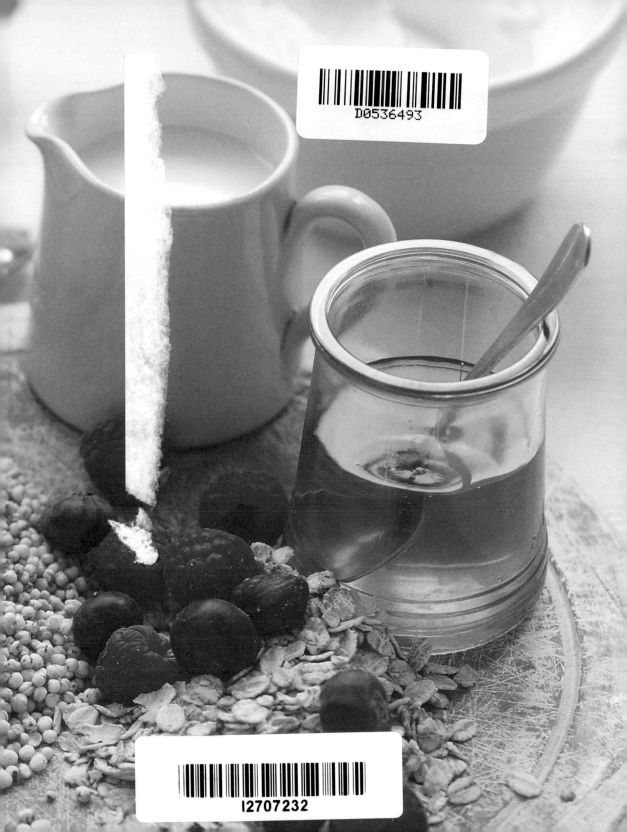

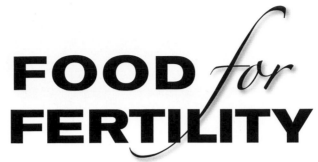

FOOD for FERTILITY

THE CONCEPTION AND PREGNANCY COOKBOOK

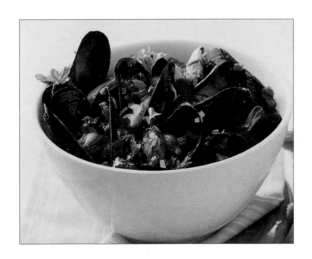

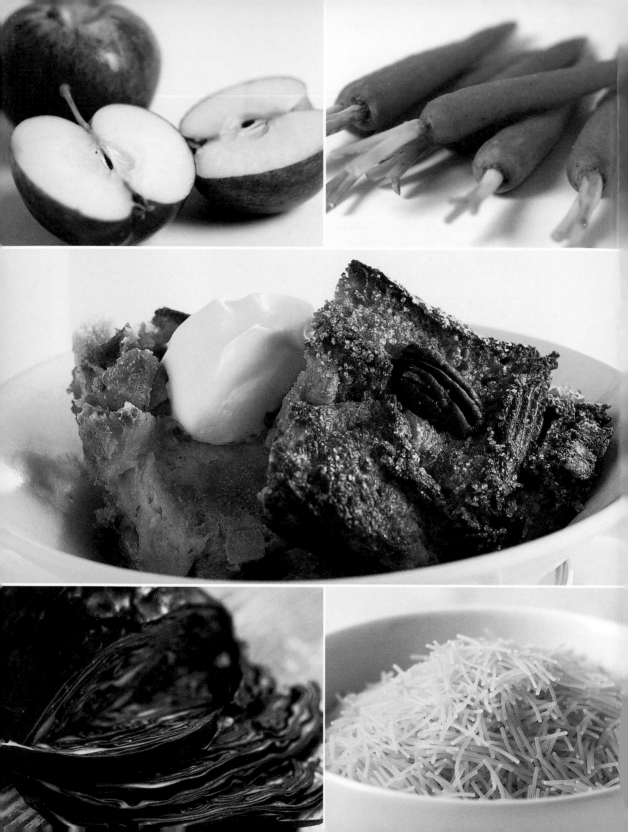

FOOD *for* FERTILITY

THE CONCEPTION AND PREGNANCY COOKBOOK

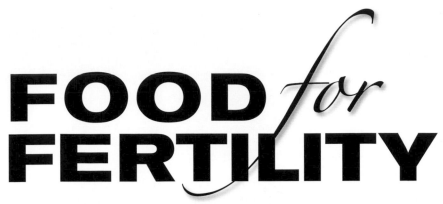

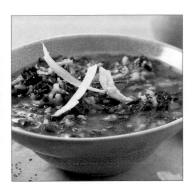
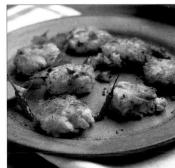
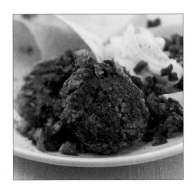

50 nutrient-packed recipes for pre-conception,
pregnancy and breastfeeding

Katherine Burke

LORENZ BOOKS

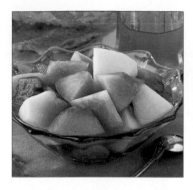
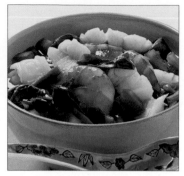
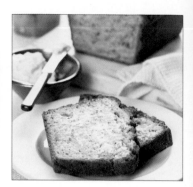
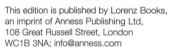

This edition is published by Lorenz Books, an imprint of Anness Publishing Ltd, 108 Great Russell Street, London WC1B 3NA; info@anness.com

www.lorenzbooks.com;
www.annesspublishing.com

If you like the images in this book and would like to investigate using them for publishing, promotions or advertising, please visit our website www.practicalpictures.com for more information.

A CIP catalogue record for this book is available from the British Library.

Publisher: Joanna Lorenz
Editor: Lucy Doncaster
Introduction: Katherine Burke, with additional text by Judy More (pp20–21)
Recipes: Catherine Atkinson, Alex Barker, Jacqueline Clark, Trisha Davies, Joanna Farrow, Brian Glover, Nicola Graimes, Deh-Ta Hsiung, Sally Mansfield, Jane Milton, Jennie Shapter, Kate Whiteman and Jeni Wright
Photography: Janine Hosegood, with additional pictures by Nicky Dowey, Ian Garlick, Michelle Garrett, Amanda Heywood, Dave Jordan, William Lingwood, Thomas Odulate, Simon Smith and Sam Stowell; Tony Stone Images (pp6 and 7)
Designer: Nigel Partridge
Production Controller: Pirong Wang

COOK'S NOTES

Bracketed terms are intended for American readers.

For all recipes, quantities are given in both metric and imperial measures and, where appropriate, in standard cups and spoons. Follow one set, but not a mixture, because they are not interchangeable.

Standard spoon and cup measures are level. 1 tsp = 5ml, 1 tbsp = 15ml, 1 cup = 250ml/8fl oz.

Australian standard tablespoons are 20ml. Australian readers should use 3 tsp in place of 1 tbsp for measuring small quantities of gelatine, flour, salt, etc.

American pints are 16fl oz/2 cups. American readers should use 20fl oz/2.5 cups in place of 1 pint when measuring liquids.

Electric oven temperatures in this book are for conventional ovens. When using a fan oven, the temperature will probably need to be reduced by about 10–20°C/20–40°F. Since ovens vary, you should check with your manufacturer's instruction book for guidance.

The nutritional analysis given for each recipe is calculated per portion (i.e. serving or item), unless otherwise stated. If the recipe gives a range, such as Serves 4–6, then the nutritional analysis will be for the smaller portion size, i.e. 6 servings. Measurements for sodium do not include salt added to taste.

Medium (US large) eggs are used unless otherwise stated.

PUBLISHER'S NOTE

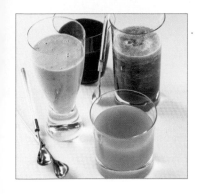
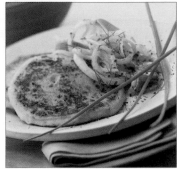
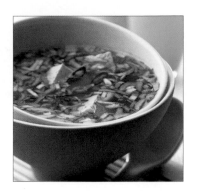

CONTENTS

Introduction

Bringing a new life into the world is probably one of the most exciting things you will ever do. The thought of being entrusted with the health and well-being of another person and nurturing them from being a tiny helpless baby into a fully grown young man or woman is wonderful. It is also a big responsibility, that can at times be daunting, so it's important to think about the practical, as well as the emotional, issues involved. Planning ahead will make it easier for you to cope with parenthood when your baby arrives.

Becoming Parents

As well as being thrilled and excited about the prospect of having a baby and becoming parents, it is also quite natural to have fears or concerns about what the future will hold. Many people worry about whether they will bond with their child; whether they will be good parents; how they will manage financially; and how they will cope with the inevitable changes in their lifestyle.

Understanding the mixed feelings about these impending changes is a natural part of expecting a baby. Talking about your hopes and fears is an important aspect of preparing for parenthood and can actually become part of the fun of planning for a family. Anticipating the adjustments you will need to make, such as having greater financial commitments or going out a little less, will help you to cope with the changes when they face you.

Moving Closer

As well as making plans for your new role as parents, it is also important to think about your relationship with your partner. In the excitement of focussing on a first baby, it is easy to neglect your own personal needs.

Pregnancy can often be a confusing time for men, with uncertainties about what their partner is experiencing and how their relationship may change after the birth. Talking about these issues will help you grow closer to your partner and will help you to build a strong relationship with your baby once it is born.

Men usually want to be involved right from the early stages of their baby's life, but beforehand they may have doubts about how to do this, and what being a good father means. Talking about fatherhood and the initial stages of

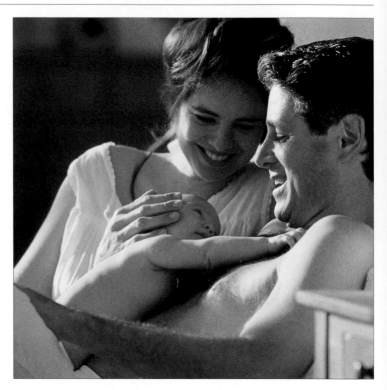

Above: Talking about parenthood during pregnancy will help you and your partner to bond with your baby and maintain a strong relationship with each other.

being new parents will ensure that you are both ready to bond with the baby and share the pressures as well as the pleasures that will come when your son or daughter arrives.

It is perfectly normal to stop being sexual for a while in late pregnancy and for a few months after the baby is born. It is important to remember that this does not mean you no longer love each other, or that you are no longer attracted to

each other. Be close and caring during this time, so that you are ready to start your sex life as soon as it feels right for both of you.

Sex is not the only issue after your baby is born. New mothers often feel exhausted, lonely and isolated when they are looking after the baby at home all day. At the same time, men can often feel rejected and marginalized because the baby comes first. Being aware of these common reactions means that you will be able to understand the situation if it occurs and should help you to avoid neglecting your partner's feelings or needs, or your relationship.

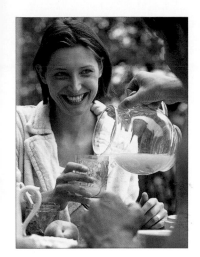

Above: A healthy, balanced diet makes sense at any time, but is especially important when you are pregnant or trying to conceive.

Practical Planning

Thinking about the practical issues before the birth will help you to relax and feel confident about coping with a new baby.

Child Care

Consider the options and decide who will look after baby and for how long. If you and your partner work, one of you may choose to stay off work permanently, or for only a year or so. Alternatively, you may both return to work after a few months, leaving baby with a child minder or at the nursery.

Taking Time Out

Discuss ways of having time off from being doting parents. Grandparents or a close friend may stay with your baby while you spend some time on your own. This may be for an hour at first, then build up to a whole evening once you feel comfortable leaving your baby.

Money Matters

Having a child is often hard on the finances. If you can, it is worth trying to save before the birth.

Thinking About Your Health

One of the greatest ways to give your child the best start in life is to make sure you and your partner are in great shape. Scientists have discovered that much of our adult health is governed by influences before we were born. Problems in later life, such as high blood pressure, diabetes and heart disease, are linked to low birth weight.

Both parents' diets, general health, fitness and environment can have an enormous impact on the health of their offspring. Eating a well-balanced diet before and during pregnancy is vital to your baby's health. The advice and recipes you will find in this book are designed to take you through the stages of pre-conception, pregnancy and breastfeeding to give your baby the best chances in life. Men can raise their sperm counts and ensure they become fit and active fathers by giving up smoking,

Below: Getting involved from the very first stages of pregnancy can help new fathers develop a close bond with their baby.

cutting down on alcohol and reducing their exposure to pesticides and other toxins. These simple lifestyle changes can help to boost male fertility, promote a healthy pregnancy and may help to reduce the risk of miscarriage.

It is natural for women, in particular, to be conscious of factors that could be harmful to the baby while it is developing in the womb. However, it is important not to overreact and to constantly feel guilty or worried about what you do and what you eat. The important thing is to pick out the healthy foods you enjoy without forcing yourself to eat food you hate. Making two simple changes to your diet – eating plenty of oily fish and avoiding any type of fast food – can make an impact on the health of your baby.

Taking regular exercise is important for both parents and will help you cope with all the exciting, and sometimes tiring, changes that lie ahead.

Being happy, following a healthy lifestyle and enjoying your pregnancy throughout all the stages will help you to produce a healthy, lively baby.

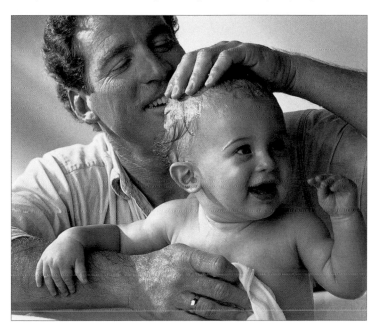

Understanding fertility

Taking a little time to find out about how your body works and what can affect your fertility can be invaluable when you are trying to conceive. As well as external factors, such as diet and lifestyle, men's and women's fertility is also governed by their biology. Women are tied to a monthly cycle, during which they are only fertile for a short time, while men produce a regular supply of sperm.

Fertility and conception are complex but the good news is that four in five couples will conceive within a year if they make love several times a week. Male and female fertility declines with age, more so for women from their mid-thirties, but you can improve your chances of conception by cleaning up your diet and lifestyle and making love more often at the woman's most fertile time. It is best to have sex every 2–3 days as this will allow time for the sperm count to recover.

Female Fertility

The ovaries are similar in size to large grapes and there is one on either side of the womb, near the Fallopian tubes. They produce eggs and the hormones oestrogen and progesterone. These hormones govern a woman's monthly cycle under the guidance of two brain hormones, the luteinising hormone and follicle stimulating hormone. Each month an egg ripens in one of the ovaries and is released, then wafted down the Fallopian tube towards the womb – this process is known as ovulation.

Before ovulation the ovaries produce increasing amounts of oestrogen, which stimulates the lining of the womb to thicken. The cervix also produces clear, stretchy mucus for the sperm to feed on, which allows them to survive for up to 5 days.

After the egg is released from a follicle on the ovary, the follicle starts to produce progesterone, which raises the body temperature.

The woman's egg can survive in the Fallopian fluid for approximately 12–24 hours. If the egg is not fertilized during this time, the progesterone levels fall and the lining of the womb shrinks, dies and is finally shed as a period 14 days later. The unfertilized egg is shed along with the womb lining.

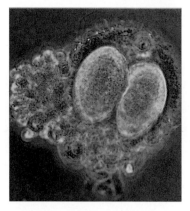

Above: Every baby starts its life as a fertilized egg, which multiplies again and again to develop into the embryo.

When you are Most Fertile

By taking note of the physical changes that occur in your body during your monthly cycle, it is possible to work out when you are at your most fertile. Because sperm can survive for 3–4 days inside a woman's body, a woman can conceive if she has sex during the 5 days following her period when her vagina no longer feels dry. The mucus becomes clear and stretchy several days before you ovulate. At the same time you can sometimes feel the neck of the womb rise and soften and you may feel sexier. Some women also notice ovulation pain – a twinge low down and to one side of their abdomen.

As well as being aware of the changes in the vagina and cervical mucus, your temperature can also indicate when you are fertile, as it rises slightly after ovulation. Use the chart on the opposite page to work out when you are most fertile, by recording the changes that occur to your body. Start from the first day of your period and take your temperature every morning before you get out of bed. Normal body temperature is about 37°C/98.6°F, but it rises by around 0.2°C/0.36°F after ovulation. It stays at this slightly higher temperature for 14 days until your period. If your body remains at the higher temperature for more than 20 days, it is more than likely that you are pregnant.

It usually takes a few months of charting to find the pattern in your cycle. Some women find the watching and waiting stressful, especially as it is not necessarily easy to see the pattern on your own. Contacting a natural family planning organization and arranging to see a fertility adviser can be helpful if you are not having much success.

Another way to check when you are at your most fertile is to use an ovulation kit. These are designed for testing urine and detect the rise in luteinising hormone just before ovulation. If one of these tests indicates a rise in the hormone in your urine sample, having sex within 24 hours of taking the test will increase your chances of conception. Follow the manufacturer's instructions carefully for using the kit.

If You Don't Conceive Straight Away

If you and your partner have both taken stock of your lifestyle and diet, and still have not conceived after a year of trying, you may decide to seek medical advice or have fertility checks. Women over 36 should see their doctor sooner.

Even without treatment, about one in three couples who could not conceive in the first year succeed in the second, so don't feel that all is lost if you don't fall pregnant after the first few attempts.

Charting Your Fertile Phase

Date																																			
Day of cycle	1	2	3	4	5	6	7	8	9	10	11	12	13	14	15	16	17	18	19	20	21	22	23	24	25	26	27	28	29	30	31	32	33	34	35
Temperature C / F																																			
Background signals																																			
Vaginal fluids																																			
Cervix changes																																			

Temperature scale (°C / °F):
38.0 / 99.0
37.0 / 98.0
36.0 / 97.0

Male Fertility

Sperm start off as primitive sperm cells that divide to produce young sperm. These grow in nourishment cells until their tails are partially formed. Then they move to a coil of tubes located on top of the testes. The sperm swim up a tube called the vas deferens, ready to be released. This all takes 70–100 days.

Male Fertility Boosters

There are several steps a man can take to improve his sperm count:

- Sperm are sensitive to heat and do not survive overheating. Wear loose boxer shorts instead of tight pants to keep the testes cool, and take showers instead of soaking in hot baths.
- Ginseng can help to increase sperm count and sperm motility.

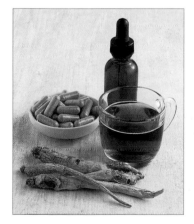

Above: Ginseng can increase sperm count and sperm motility as well as increasing energy levels.

Above: Use this chart to help establish when you are at your most fertile.

Conception

After ejaculation, about 100 sperm survive the journey through the womb to the Fallopian tubes and the egg. The sperm release an enzyme that breaks down the membrane that surrounds the egg until one sperm head successfully enters the egg.

The genetic material from the sperm and egg fuse and the fertilized egg is wafted down the Fallopian tube until, about a week after ovulation, it reaches the womb. After fertilization, the egg begins to divide. By the time a fertilized egg reaches the womb, it has become a ball of cells, which implants itself in the walls of the womb.

Getting ready for conception

To give your baby the best chances in life, try to clean up your diet and lifestyle four months before you try to conceive. Getting into peak physical condition well before you conceive gives both eggs and sperm time to recover from the wear and tear caused by modern living. Eggs are most vulnerable about 100 days before they are released and sperm are fragile for 3½ months before they mature. The human body is very resilient and can take just a few months to get into shape. A few small changes can go a long way towards undoing damage caused by poor diet, lack of exercise or overindulgence.

Improving Your Lifestyle

Getting ready for conception means eating a healthy, well-balanced diet, taking regular exercise and giving up bad habits such as smoking.

Make an effort to move about frequently during the day and aim to do some energetic walking, cycling or structured exercise at least three times every week.

Stop smoking and reduce your consumption of alcohol and caffeine. Do not use any recreational drugs.

The Benefits of Giving up Cigarettes and Alcohol

Giving up smoking improves both male and female fertility. Smoking by either parent increases the risk of miscarriage and birth defects. It is never too late to stop smoking and within 3 months the damage can be reversed. Set a date to give up and stick to it. If you both smoke,

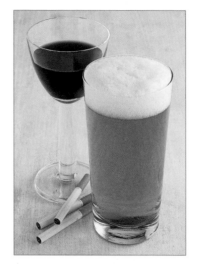

support each other and give up together. Remember to tell everyone you know so that they will help you with the new regime. Think about all the money you will save and plan a treat as a reward.

Alcohol can also affect fertility. Even a couple of drinks a day lowers male and female fertility while raising the chances of miscarriage. Ideally, men should avoid regular drinking for at least 3 months before conception. Women should also give up drinking alcohol, especially from day 10 of the cycle, when the egg is at its most vulnerable.

Above: To boost your combined fertility and reduce the risk of miscarriage, stop smoking and cut down on alcohol.

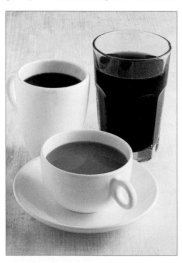

Left: Prospective mothers should steer clear of drinks containing caffeine, as these can affect their chances of a healthy pregnancy.

Your Fertile Weight

Being overweight can affect male fertility and being underweight can affect female fertility. Women usually have to weigh at least 44.5kg/98lb/7 stone before they are fertile because the body has to carry a certain amount of fat for the brain to stimulate ovulation. To ensure optimum fertility, a woman's BMI (Body Mass Index) should be 25. Below 20 is underweight and above 30 is obese. The normal range is 20–25. Use the formula below to calculate your BMI:

$$\frac{\text{weight (kg)}}{\text{height (m)} \times \text{height (m)}}$$

Reducing the Risk of Miscarriage

Many miscarriages are caused by a one-off chromosomal abnormality in the baby. If you are particularly worried about miscarriage, the following advice for both potential parents may reduce the risk.

• Cut out coffee and other caffeinated drinks and medication containing caffeine, such as cold and flu remedies. In a vulnerable individual, just one to three cups of coffee a day can double the risk of losing the baby.

• Do not drink or smoke.

• If you are very overweight, talk to your doctor about eating sensibly to lose the excess.

• Selenium is thought to protect sperm, eggs and the baby against chromosomal damage that is often responsible for miscarriages. Zinc is believed to play a similar role.

Avoid Chemicals That May Harm Your Baby

We all have 300–500 synthetic chemicals in our body, acquired from pesticides and as by-products of incineration. Potentially the most harmful are polychlorinated chemicals such as PCBs (Polychlorinated Biphenyls), which are now banned in the United States, and dioxins. These oestrogen-mimicking chemicals dissolve in our fat, to be passed on to our children through the placenta and breast milk. The body has difficulty in getting rid of these chemicals because the liver cannot break them down.

Why Polychlorinated Chemicals are Harmful

Polychlorinated chemicals have been linked to cancer as well as problems with the immune system and reproduction. Children exposed to high levels of dioxins in the womb tend to have softer teeth and lower IQs than their exposure-free classmates.

How to Avoid Polychlorinated Chemicals

Eating organic food should reduce exposure to hormone-disrupting chemicals. The following foods are low in these chemicals:
- Fruits, vegetables and other plant produce, such as beans and pulses.
- Deep-water sea fish, such as herring, mackerel and sardines.
- Meat, which has been trimmed of fat. You may also prefer to buy paper products, such as tea bags, coffee filter papers, that have not been bleached with chlorine, including tampons. Glass bottles are preferable to paper cartons.

Avoiding Other Everyday Chemicals and Radiation

You should also try to limit your exposure to chemicals that can be found in many everyday products. These chemicals, as well as radiation, can lead to a reduction in fertility.
- Use a water filter if you are worried about the quality of your water supply.

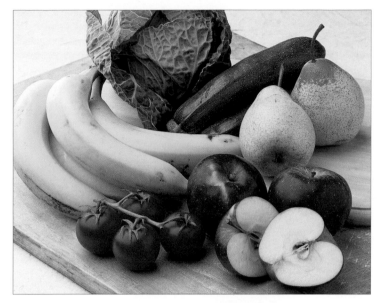

Above: Whenever you can, eat organic fruit and vegetables rather than conventionally produced ones as they contain fewer of the harmful chemicals that can affect your unborn child.

The water company will be able to check contaminant levels. If you live in an old house, check the plumbing and have any lead pipes replaced.
- Solvents used in paints, paint strippers and varnishes can be harmful, so any home improvements should, if possible, be delayed. When stripping paintwork, always wear protective clothing, including a face mask and hair protector. If you need to paint, try to finish several months before you stop using contraception.
- Avoid medical X-rays .
- Couples, especially women, should avoid using wood preservatives, pesticides, head-lice shampoos and flea sprays near the time of conception; these products should also be avoided by pregnant women. At high exposure levels, many of these products can impair your fertility and cause impotence, miscarriage or birth defects.

Visit Your Doctor

Take time to have a health review. If you or your partner are on long-term medication, it is worth reviewing the options with your doctor. Cut down on medication for minor ailments.

Women should go for a general health check. The doctor or nurse will check your blood pressure, and give you a cervical smear test, if you are due for one, and a breast examination. Ask them to check your blood group and, if you are rhesus negative, ask your doctor about how you will be treated during the birth or if you were to bleed during the pregnancy. It may be worth asking to have a test to check for diabetes.

Women should also check their immunity to rubella and toxoplasmosis. If necessary arrange a vaccination. Wait 3 months before trying to conceive.

Seek medical advice if you have any abnormal discharge or a condition such as cystitis or thrush.

If you or your partner are at risk of a sexually transmitted infection, you should both go to a genito-urinary clinic and complete any treatment before trying to conceive.

Positive eating for conception

As well as cleaning up your lifestyle, plan about four months of positive eating in readiness for conception. A well-balanced diet for men and women is one of the keys to producing a healthy baby. Include wholegrain ingredients and at least five portions of fruit and vegetables a day. Where available, organic foods are best because they contain fewer pesticides than conventionally produced foods.

Eating a Balanced Diet

A healthy diet is full of variety. It is packed with fruit and vegetables and includes starchy carbohydrate, whole-foods, such as unprocessed grains and pulses, and protein. Carbohydrates should make up around 50 per cent of your daily diet, which should also include five or more portions of vegetables and fruit, some meat, fish or other protein foods, and three servings of low-fat dairy foods, such as milk, yogurt or cheese. Foods that are high in fat and sugar, such as cakes and biscuits, should be eaten only occasionally.

You should eat regular meals three times a day, including at least one main meal. Try not to skip meals.

Below: Eating a variety of foods will help to provide your body with all the nutrients it needs for conception.

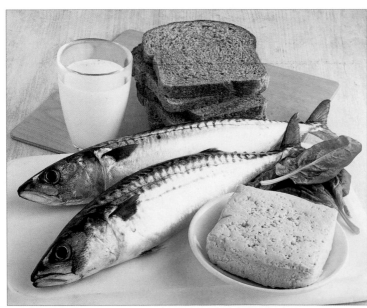

Foods for Conception

As well as following the guidelines for a healthy, balanced diet, you should also eat plenty of the following foods and nutrients to prepare for conception:

- Focus on foods rich in folic acid, such as leafy green vegetables, broccoli, Brussels sprouts, oranges, eggs, fortified breakfast cereals, pulses, wheatgerm and cashew nuts.
- Eat at least 115g/4oz protein foods a day, such as fish, poultry or meat. If you are vegetarian, aim for at least 350g/12oz high-protein foods such as beans, nuts and pulses.
- Include calcium-rich foods, such as dairy products, fish in which the bones are eaten like canned sardines, and beancurd (tofu).
- Try to eat at least 1 portion of oily fish, such as mackerel, sardines, herring or tuna, a week.

- Use good-quality vegetable oils, such as cold-pressed olive oil, to boost your intake of essential fatty acids.
- Use unhydrogenated olive oil margarines, made by new methods, rather than butter, which is high in saturated fats.
- Eat several slices of wholemeal (whole-wheat) bread a day as it provides good supplies of B vitamins and trace elements, such as magnesium, selenium and zinc.

Nutrients to Boost Fertility

Researchers are investigating the use of vitamin E as a supplement to boost fertility; high-quality sperm contains more vitamin E than poor-quality sperm. It may also correct impotence and boost libido. Vitamin E is also needed to prevent polyunsaturated vegetable oils in the diet being oxidized in the body. Men and women need about 10mg of vitamin E per day, although 4–5 times that amount is still considered healthy. Good sources of vitamin E include:

- 50g/2oz/½ cup hazelnuts or almonds supplies 14mg of vitamin E. Other nuts are also good sources, including peanuts and pine nuts.
- 30ml/2 tbsp sunflower seeds provides 7mg. Other good sources include sunflower oil and olive oil.
- 100g/3¾oz/¾ cup wheatgerm provides 22mg.
- Sweet potatoes and avocados contain useful amounts.

Another nutrient thought to boost fertility is the antioxidant selenium. Lack of selenium may lead to infertility in men and possibly miscarriage in women. It is also believed to help protect DNA from damage. The recommended daily intake of selenium varies between 60–75µg. Selenium is transferred to produce from the soil in which it is grown – soil in the

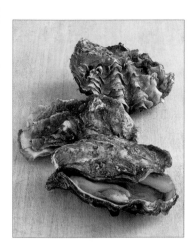

Above: Oysters, which have been famed as aphrodisiacs for centuries, are rich in the mineral zinc, which is thought to promote healthy sperm.

poisoning than cooked oysters.)
• 100g/3¾oz crab, topside of beef or leg of lamb provides 5.5mg.
• 100g/3¾oz sardines provides 3mg.
• Dairy products, Brazil nuts, lentils and sunflower seeds.

Foods to Avoid
Although some foods are better than others, most "natural" or unprocessed foods will not harm you if they are eaten in the right proportion. Processed products are the ones to avoid because they are often low in protein and other essential nutrients but tend to be high in fat, especially unhealthy saturated fats, refined carbohydrates and salt.

Right: Wheatgerm, almonds and hazelnuts are rich in vitamin E, which is thought to boost fertility and help impotence.

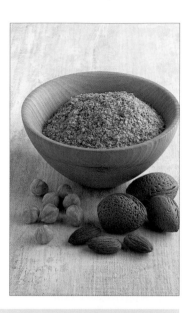

USA is richer in selenium than UK soil, and areas of Brazil have some of the most selenium-rich soils in the world.

Just two Brazil nuts will provide a day's supply of selenium. Other good sources include seafood, especially mackerel and herring, wheatgerm, sunflower seeds and eggs. In the United States, where the soil is particularly rich in selenium, wholemeal (whole-wheat) flour is also a good source.

Foods to Make You Frisky
Many foods traditionally reputed to be aphrodisiacs are rich in nutrients that are thought to promote fertility, particularly zinc, which is needed for a good sperm count and healthy development of the foetus. The best source of zinc is seafood, particularly oysters, which contain large amounts of this nutrient. (Avoid shellfish during pregnancy as there is a slight risk of food poisoning.) The recommended daily intake of zinc varies between 7–15mg, with men needing slightly more. Mothers-to-be who do not eat enough zinc tend to give birth to smaller babies. Good sources include:
• Six cooked oysters provide 24mg. (Raw oysters carry a higher risk of food

Nutritional Supplements
In addition to eating the right balance of foods, many people choose to take nutritional supplements to ensure they receive all the nutrients that are needed for conception and a healthy pregnancy.

Seek advice from a doctor before taking supplements during pregnancy.

Before Pregnancy
You and your partner may wish to take a multivitamin and mineral supplement specially designed for pre-conception. This should contain vitamin B_{12} and the B vitamin, folic acid, as both help to protect against neural tube defects, such as spina bifida, plus iron, zinc and beta-carotene, the safe form of vitamin A. Do not take supplements containing vitamin A (retinol), which can be harmful in pregnancy.

A vegan diet can often be low in certain nutrients, such as vitamin B_{12}, iron and calcium. Women who are vegans may therefore wish to supplement their diet with extra doses of these nutrients for a few months before conception.

During Pregnancy
Taking large doses of vitamins during pregnancy can be dangerous and is not recommended. It is, however, recommended that pregnant women take a 400µg daily dose of folic acid, making a total daily intake of 600µg; and a vitamin D supplement to make up a total daily intake of 10mg.

Vegetarians may want to take a Vitamin B_{12} supplement until the second trimester, as this nutrient is hard to obtain from a vegetarian diet.

Additional iron should not be required as the body becomes more efficient at absorbing nutrients during pregnancy and iron is not lost through menstrual bleeding, which ceases during pregnancy. Iron supplements at high doses may cause constipation, a common problem in pregnancy, so make sure you do not take more than 100% of the RDA.

Cod liver oil contains too much vitamin A, which may harm the developing baby. Do not take supplements containing more than 100% of the RDA of vitamin A.

Eating in early pregnancy

When you become pregnant, your body will go through some fairly major changes. The hormones that are released to keep your pregnancy going can affect the way you feel, making you tired and affecting your emotions and digestion. The changes occurring to your body may also affect your appetite, but it is vitally important to continue to eat a healthy diet during the first three months.

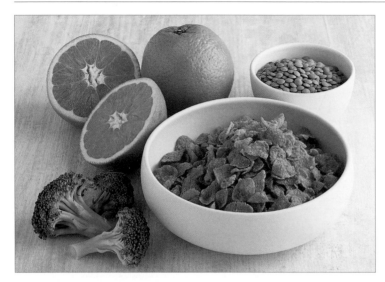

It is normal to gain about 3.6kg/8lb in the first 20 weeks of pregnancy. Eat plenty of oily fish, lean meat and poultry, especially free-range chicken, free-range eggs, nuts, beans, lentils and seeds. Also aim to eat plenty of fruit and vegetables, including at least one portion of leafy green vegetables a day, plus wheatgerm, wholemeal (whole-wheat) bread and fortified breakfast cereals.

Nutrients for Your Baby

The B vitamins are essential for your baby's development during the first 3 months of pregnancy. Folic acid, one of the B vitamins, is very important for making new cells and vitamin B_{12} is needed to produce the protective coating around nerves. Together, folic acid and vitamin B_{12} make healthy red blood cells and help to protect your baby from neural tube defects, such as spina bifida, which are abnormalities caused by the brain and spinal cord failing to develop properly in the womb.

Above: Broccoli, oranges, fortified cereals and lentils contain folic acid.

Getting Enough Folic Acid

The recommended daily intake of folic acid is 600µg while you are trying to conceive and until the 12th week of pregnancy. If you are taking a 400µg supplement, your diet should provide the remaining 200µg.

Good sources include:
• Vegetables such as Brussels sprouts, spinach, broccoli, French (green) beans, artichokes, cauliflower, asparagus and sweetcorn. Folic acid is water soluble, so use the cooking water from vegetables in soups or sauces.
• Nuts, such as peanuts, hazelnuts, and walnuts.
• Fortified breakfast cereals usually provide 100µg folic acid per portion (check the information on the packet).
• 115g/4oz boiled lentils provides 180µg folic acid.
• 1 orange provides 50µg folic acid.

Getting Enough Vitamin B₁₂

The recommended daily intake of vitamin B_{12} for pregnant women varies from 1.5µg–2.6µg.

Good sources include kidneys, tuna and other oily fish, eggs and some fortified breakfast cereals.
• 50g/2oz lamb's kidney contains 45µg of vitamin B_{12}.
• 75g/3oz canned tuna in water contains 2.5µg.
• 1 egg provides 0.75µg and free-range eggs over 25 per cent more.
Vegan sources include fortified soya products and spirulina, a freshwater algae supplement.

Easing Morning Sickness

When you first become pregnant, your saliva becomes more acidic, which may make you feel queasy. About seven in ten pregnant women are affected by morning sickness, which is thought to be related to the radical changes in hormone levels early in pregnancy.

Below: Drink plenty of orange juice, as it helps the body to absorb valuable folic acid needed for your growing baby.

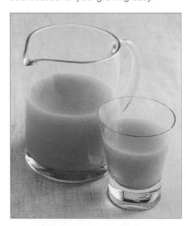

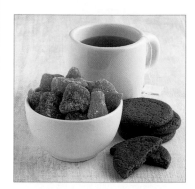

Above: Combat morning sickness by sipping ginger tea or eating crystallized ginger and gingernuts (gingersnaps).

An empty stomach can make nausea worse, so make sure you eat little and often. When you do not feel like a meal, eat a nutritious snack rather than a high-fat processed food or something sugary. Try oat cakes, crackers, bananas, fruit buns, low-fat rice pudding, yogurts, breakfast cereals with skimmed (low-fat) milk, toast, crispbreads, bread or fresh fruit milkshakes.

Herb teas containing chamomile, fennel or lemon balm help to reduce nausea, as does ginger, so try drinking ginger tea, ginger ale, ginger beer or eating preserved ginger or ginger-flavoured biscuits (cookies).

Avoid fatty, spicy dishes or strongly flavoured foods as these can make you feel more nauseous.

It's not only foods that can combat nausea. There is also good evidence that some alternative therapies, such as acupuncture, may help to quell feelings of sickness.

Fluids
It is very important to drink plenty of fluids. During pregnancy your total body water content increases by about 4 litres/7 pints, so try to drink at least 8 glasses of fluid a day, preferably water. You can also drink fruit juice, milk, herbal or fruit teas or uncaffeinated coffee substitutes, such as *Barley Cup*.

Foods to Limit
There is nothing wrong with the occasional indulgence, but do not fill up on foods that have poor nutritional value. Instead, concentrate on eating the healthy, nutritious foods.
- Sweets, cakes and sugar are low in nutrients. Having a dessert or a small piece of chocolate after a nutritious meal is fine, but try to eat fruit or fruit-based desserts instead of rich, high-fat, high-sugar puddings.
- Limit coffee, tea, colas, chocolate and other caffeinated food and drinks. Tea also contains tannin, which inhibits iron absorption.
- Try not to eat too much processed food. Always read the labels and try to avoid foods containing preservatives, colourings and other additives.

Foods to Avoid
There are several food-borne infections that can be dangerous for pregnant women and their developing baby. Listeriosis is a rare flu-like illness caused by the harmful listeria bacteria. It can cause miscarriage, stillbirth or severe illness in the newborn baby.

Toxoplasmosis is also a rare flu-like illness caused by a parasite found in cat faeces, raw meat and, occasionally, goat's milk. In rare cases it can cross the placenta, causing brain damage and blindness. Salmonella is a type of food poisoning that will make you feel dreadful but should not harm your unborn baby.

Foods that carry the risk of these infections and which should be avoided include:
- Pâtés, except canned pâtés, which may contain listeria.
- Brie, Camembert and other cheeses with a similar soft white rind, may contain listeria; as may blue-veined cheeses such as Stilton. These cheeses can, however, be eaten when cooked, for example as part of a hot dish.
- Sheep and goat products sometimes carry listeria, so they are only safe if they are made from pasteurized milk.
- Soft ice cream from a machine may

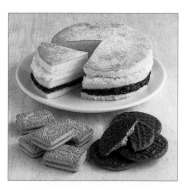

Above: Cut down on fresh cream cakes and rich biscuits as they are high in trans fatty acids.

contain listeria due to poor hygiene. Ice cream from a tub should be safe.
- Raw or undercooked meat, poultry and eggs may contain salmonella. Avoid dishes such as soft-boiled eggs, chilled soufflés or home-made mayonnaise.
- Raw shellfish, such as oysters, should be avoided in pregnancy, as they carry a risk of food poisoning.

Liver and liver products, such as pâté, should also be avoided during pregnancy. They can contain large amounts of vitamin A, which has been linked to formation of cleft palate when eaten in large doses.

Avoid Alcohol
There is no safe drinking limit during pregnancy. Try to abstain from alcohol completely in the first 3 months.

Cheeses That are Safe to Eat When Pregnant
Although unpasteurized cheeses should be avoided, there are still plenty that can be eaten, including hard cow's cheeses, such as Cheddar, Cheshire and Parmesan. Mozzarella is good for salads. Cottage cheese can be included. Pasteurized sheep's and goat's cheeses are acceptable.

Vital foods for your second trimester

By the end of your third month of pregnancy, your appetite and energy levels should be returning to normal and you are probably fitter than ever and looking radiant. You should continue to eat normally rather than piling your plate with double portions (it is a myth that you have to 'eat for two'). During months four to six, your baby's pancreas is developing and you will need lots of zinc to help it form properly. You also need to prepare for the growth spurt in your baby's brain at the end of the second trimester.

Vital Nutrients for Foetal Growth

A baby needs varying types of nutrients in the different stages of its development. During the second trimester, the baby's pancreas is at a critical stage of development. Make sure you eat plenty of zinc-rich foods, such as red meat, spinach and sunflower seeds during this time, as this nutrient is essential for proper development of the pancreas.

You also need to prepare for the growth spurt in your baby's brain that will occur from around the sixth month. In the final three months of pregnancy the baby's brain will grow rapidly (at birth it will be 25 per cent of the size of an adult brain). The brain is made up of 60 per cent fat, half of which takes the form of DHA (docosahexaenoic acid), a long chain omega-3 fatty acid.

You need to eat plenty of these essential fatty acids, which are found in oily fish, as they are vital for the developing baby's brain, retina and nervous system. They may also help to produce a bigger baby and reduce the chances of premature birth.

It is recommended that a good proportion of oily fish is eaten in a normal healthy diet and this becomes more important during pregnancy. Aim to eat at least one portion of oily fish a week, such as kippers, pilchards or mackerel.

Below: Eating one portion of oily fish a week is not just good for a mother-to-be; it also benefits her baby.

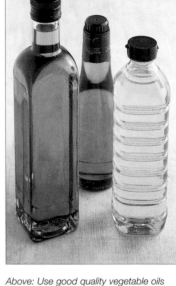

Above: Use good quality vegetable oils for cooking, such as cold-pressed olive oil, sunflower oil and walnut oil.

Canned sardines and salmon are also good sources of omega-3 fatty acids. Non-fish sources of this vital nutrient include soya beans, beancurd (tofu), almonds, walnuts, hazelnuts, safflower and sunflower seeds and their oils, rapeseed oil, eggs and lean game.

To make the most of omega-3 fatty acids found in fish, eat lots of foods rich in antioxidants such as vitamins C and E, selenium and carotenoids. These will protect the delicate fish oils from destruction by oxidation.

Sources of antioxidants in fresh food include:
• Kiwi fruit and fresh strawberries provide vitamin C.

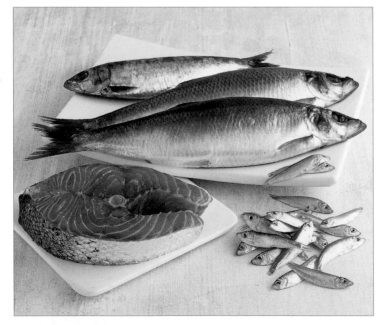

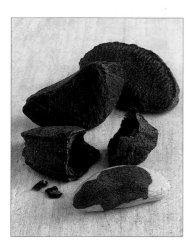

Above: Brazil nuts are a very good source of selenium, which helps to protect valuable fish oils and their nutrients from destruction by oxidation.

- Avocados and nuts provide vitamin E.
- Peppers provide vitamin C and carotenoids. Carotenoids are also found in other brightly coloured vegetables and fruit, such as carrots, tomatoes, mangoes and papayas.
- Brazil nuts, grown in Brazil, provide rich supplies of selenium.

If you do not eat fish, you might want to try fish oil supplements made from the flesh of oily fish. Do not use fish liver oils during pregnancy, as they may contain too much vitamin A, as well as pollutants at low levels.

Foods to Ease Constipation

Constipation is a common problem for many women during pregnancy.
- Try drinking a glass of hot water first thing in the morning to get your digestive system moving. Adding a slice of lemon to it is also very refreshing.
- Improve your fibre intake by eating oats in porridge or muesli for breakfast. They contain soluble fibre, which absorbs moisture, swells and softens in the digestive tract and are less harsh on the digestive system than bran.
- Fresh apples, eaten with their peel, and cooked vegetables can help.
- Liquorice may also be good for easing constipation.

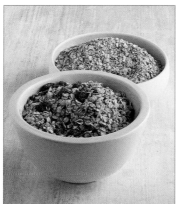

Above: Oats and foods containing oats, such as muesli, will provide plenty of soluble fibre and can ease constipation.

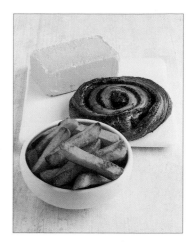

Above: Avoid Danish pastries, chips (French fries) and hydrogenated margarines as they tend to contain large amounts of unhealthy trans fatty acids.

Fats to Avoid

Although essential fatty acids are good for you and your baby, not all fats are beneficial. Unhealthy trans fatty acids, which are produced by some modern methods of food processing, should be avoided. Foods to avoid include: mass-produced cakes and cookies, all types of fast foods, such as burgers, chips (French fries) and pizza, and hydrogenated margarines.

Your total daily intake of fat should not exceed 70g and this should be mainly made up of unsaturated fats.

Food Safety and Cooking

Pay particular attention to the way you store, prepare and cook food during pregnancy.
- Check that your refrigerator is always kept at a temperature below 5°C/40° F.
- Cook or serve frozen food within 24 hours of thawing. Never refreeze foods that have been thawed.
- Do not eat any food that is past its sell-by date.

- Wash kitchen surfaces, utensils and your hands after contact with raw fish, poultry, meat or eggs. This also applies to other foods that have to be cooked before being eaten.
- Wash fruit, vegetables and pre-packed salads well, especially if they are to be eaten raw, because there is a slight risk of toxoplasmosis.
- Always reheat cooked foods or meals until they are piping hot throughout, particularly poultry dishes.

Useful Cooking Methods

How you cook food is almost as important as the nutrients they contain. Always try to choose a healthy cooking method.
- Steam oily fish rather than grilling (broiling), frying or baking as this helps to retain omega-3 fatty acids.
- Avoid frying, particularly frying repeatedly in the same oil, because this causes the oil to break down and trans fatty acids to be formed.

Eating in late pregnancy

During the final three months of pregnancy, your body will undergo even more dramatic changes as the baby continues to grow in size and develop. At this stage you will need to eat more and you will gain weight, but it is important to carry on eating the nutrients needed to keep your body in peak condition.

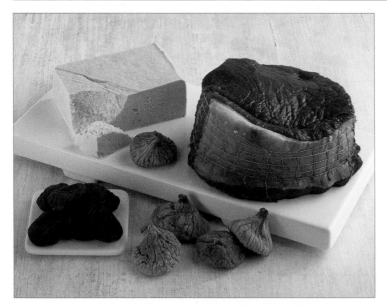

Above: Foods that provide a good source of iron include red meat, beancurd, dried figs and dried apricots.

In the last three months before birth, a pregnant woman will usually gain up to 450g/1lb per week. Her daily energy requirement will increase by about 200–300 kcalories (10–20 per cent). An average total weight gain is 12.5kg/27½lb. The baby will account for about 3.1kg/7lb and the rest goes towards the growing womb, placenta and breasts. If you gain much more than this, discuss the increase with your midwife as a very large weight gain can raise blood pressure, increase pressure on the joints and prove difficult to lose later, after the baby is born.

Anaemia in Pregnancy

Although some women develop anaemia in later in pregnancy, it is thought that this condition tends to be overdiagnosed or misdiagnosed. Towards the end of pregnancy, the blood becomes diluted and the ideal haemoglobin concentration during the last month is lower than that for a non-pregnant woman. A slightly low red cell count is a good sign of blood dilution and placental activity.

The recommended intake of iron for pregnant women varies from about 15mg to 30mg; men need about 10mg. Talk to your health adviser about whether you need supplements, and include iron-rich foods in your diet. Red meat contains haem iron, which is more accessible to the body than vegetable-based iron. The following foods are all good sources of iron:

• 75g/3oz clams provides 8mg.
• 100g/3¾oz portion of topside of beef provides 3mg.
• 100g/3¾oz beancurd (tofu) provides 1.2mg.
• 8 dried figs contain 4.5mg.
• Other good sources include fish, lentils, chickpeas, almonds, baked beans and dried apricots.

Although wholegrain flour and cereals contain a lot of iron, they also contain fibre which binds to the iron, making it less easy to absorb.

To make the most of iron, combine iron-rich foods with vitamin C-rich foods. The vitamin C will help the body to absorb iron. Try drinking a glass of orange juice with an iron-rich dish. Do not drink tea or eat dairy products for an hour before or after eating an iron-rich meal, as they inhibit iron absorption.

Heartburn

This is a common condition in late pregnancy, caused by pressure from the baby on the stomach pushing some acid up into the oesophagus. It tends to get worse when you lean forward or lie down.

• Try eating six small meals a day instead of three large ones.
• Eat slowly.
• Avoid spicy and fatty foods.

Below: Sipping chamomile and lemon balm tea can help calm the stomach and ease painful heartburn.

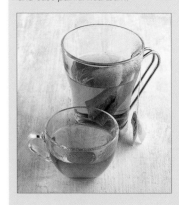

Calcium for Healthy Bones and Teeth

Eating a diet which is low in calcium during pregnancy is unlikely to have adverse effects on the baby. However, it may cause the mother long-term problems such as osteoporosis, because calcium will leach out of a pregnant woman's bones and teeth to provide sufficient for the growing foetus. To avoid calcium being lost from your bones, make sure your diet provides plenty of this nutrient.

The recommended daily intake of calcium varies from 700mg to 1200mg during pregnancy. The standard advice is to have three portions of dairy products a day – 1 glass of milk, 25g/1oz cheese or a pot of yogurt. Skimmed milk (low-fat) products provide just as much calcium as whole milk. Vitamin D helps the body to absorb calcium and can be found in oily fish, eggs, margarine and from exposure to sunlight (being outside in the fresh air, rather than sunbathing).

The following foods are good sources of calcium:
- 50g/2oz whitebait provides 350mg.
- 25g/1oz Cheddar cheese provides 200mg calcium.
- 300ml/½ pint/1¼ cups skimmed milk provides 300mg.
- 50g/2oz beancurd (tofu) provides 290mg.
- Other good sources include sardines, prawns (shrimp), white self-raising (self-rising) flour, almonds, Brazil nuts, fortified soya products and spinach.

Preventing Allergies in Your Unborn Child

There is some evidence that drinking hypo-allergenic formula milk instead of cow's milk during late pregnancy may result in the baby being less likely to develop an allergy to cow's milk, or eczema. Other studies suggest that elimination diets reduce the chances of a baby becoming allergic to the specific food excluded. However, it is best to avoid eliminating foods during pregnancy and you should do so only under the supervision of a doctor or qualified dietician.

If you or your partner suffer from allergies, avoid eating peanuts and foods containing them while pregnant and breastfeeding.

Organic Foods

If you can, try to eat organic foods before conception and throughout your pregnancy. Although they tend to cost more than conventionally produced equivalents, organic foods taste better than non-organic ones, and have higher levels of vitamins and trace elements and very low levels of chemical pesticides. Another bonus is that you don't have to peel organic fruits and vegetables, although you should always scrub them well.

According to UK figures, about 30 per cent of food contains measurable pesticide residues within the prescribed limits, about 1 per cent contains residues above the permitted levels and the rest contains no detectable residues. Some foods are particularly susceptible to retaining pesticide residue, including corned beef, carrots, spinach, lettuce, potatoes, soya, apples, bread, maize, chocolate, beer and wine.

If you are unable to buy organic foods, be sure to wash vegetables and fruit thoroughly and peel carrots, which tend to contain higher levels of pesticides than other vegetables.

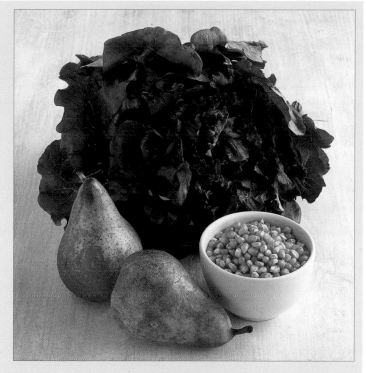

Above: Try to buy organic pears, lettuce and maize, as they tend to contain high levels of pesticide residue when grown by conventional farming methods.

Nutrients for you and your baby

Breast milk naturally provides the correct balance of nutrients and fluid that your baby needs so, in choosing to breastfeed, you are giving your baby the very best start in life. There are many advantages for both of you and it is important for you to eat regularly and well. If you choose not to breastfeed, you still need to eat the right balance of foods to help your body recover after the birth.

It's Good to Breastfeed

Breastfeeding is good for both mother and baby. Breastfed babies have fewer tummy upsets, ear infections, coughs and colds. They are also less likely to have allergies and chronic diseases such as diabetes in childhood. Breast milk is always at the right temperature, it's available on demand, there's no chance of food poisoning and it's free.

Breastfeeding is a great way to help you bond with your new baby. It can also help you get your figure back after the birth. During pregnancy, you lay down a store of fat on your thighs and hips and this is slowly used up during the first few months of breastfeeding.

Below: Breast milk provides your baby with just the right balance of nutrients.

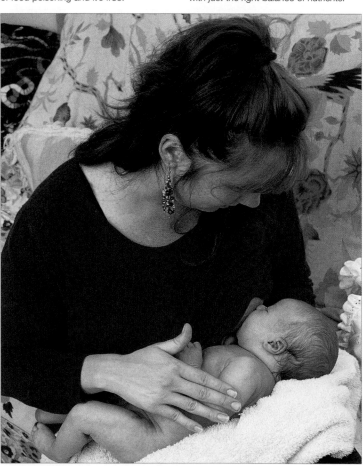

Breastfeeding Problems

Not all new mothers find breast-feeding easy to start with. It may take time for you and your baby to learn. However, with good support, advice and a little perseverance, you will succeed.

- Your breasts may become large and distended about the third day after the birth but, if you keep feeding, it should resolve within 24 hours as your supply of milk adjusts to your baby's demand.
- Sore and cracked nipples are a common problem. They may be the result of your baby being in the wrong position, so ask your health visitor or breastfeeding counsellor for advice. Another cause can be thrush in your baby's mouth, which will need medical treatment from your doctor.
- A blocked duct will feel hard and tender but will usually clear after the next feed from that breast.
- Mastitis, which is an infected blockage, will cause a hot and painful patch on your breast and may require antibiotics.

What to Eat

To ensure a good supply of milk, it is important that you rest and eat well. You need about 500 extra kcalories, an extra 11g protein, more vitamin A, C and D, B vitamins, phosphorus, zinc, copper, magnesium and selenium.

Eating a normal balanced diet with larger portions of meat, fish, pulses and milk will provide the extra protein, vitamin B_{12}, phosphorus and zinc. You will lose less calcium in your urine so eating three portions of milk, yogurt or cheese a day will be enough to replace the calcium lost

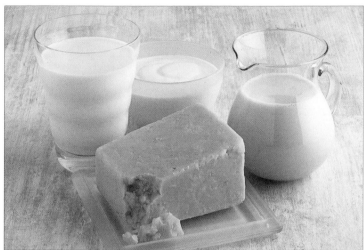

Left: Eat three portions of milk, yogurt or cheese a day to replenish calcium that is lost from the body in the weeks following birth.

Some mothers may find looking after themselves or their baby is too much, or may feel hopeless, anxious or panicky. If this occurs, it is important to seek medical advice as you may be suffering from postnatal depression, which can be dangerous if not treated.

Foods to Avoid

Avoid peanuts and unrefined peanut (groundnut) oils if you or your partner suffer from allergies, eczema or hay fever. This may prevent your baby developing a potentially serious allergy to peanuts. Some mothers believe very spicy foods and excess orange juice cause their babies to have loose stools.

Alcohol and caffeine both pass from the mother into breast milk, so limit alcoholic drinks to one with a meal and limit your intake of tea, coffee, cola drinks, energy drinks and chocolate.

from your bones during your pregnancy. If you change to higher fat milk and yogurts or treat yourself to some cream you will increase your intake of vitamins A and D. Two extra slices of wholemeal (whole-wheat) bread or an extra serving of breakfast cereal each day will provide extra B vitamins, magnesium and selenium. Having plenty of fresh fruit and some red and orange vegetables as well as dark green leafy ones will ensure you have enough vitamins A and C and folic acid.

Vitamin D is usually made by the action of sunlight on skin. If you are not going outside for some time every day or have a dark skin that you keep covered, you may need to take a supplement. The best food sources are margarine, oily fish and eggs.

You may find you become thirstier when you are breastfeeding. Make sure you drink 8–10 glasses of fluid a day, some of which should be water.

Avoiding the Baby Blues

Hormonal changes taking place in your body just after birth are usually the cause of "baby blues" during the first week of your baby's life. In the weeks following birth, while you are getting up during the night to feed your baby, you will probably become tired. This can reduce your appetite but beware of skipping meals. Regular meals and snacks will keep your blood sugar more even and you will be less likely to become irritable, lose your self-esteem or slip into mild depression, all of which can happen to new mothers.

If You Aren't Breastfeeding

The baby milks available today are made to resemble breast milk, with all the nutrients required for your baby to grow and develop normally. Care must be taken to make them up correctly to ensure the correct balance of nutrients and fluid. Always sterilize bottles and teats to make sure no bacteria harm your baby.

If you cannot breastfeed for any reason, or choose not to, getting rid of weight gained during pregnancy can be more difficult. Accept that it will take time and eat sensibly as drastic dieting, on top of tiredness from looking after your baby, may cause depression. Eat plenty of low-fat starchy foods, fruit and vegetables and exercise more.

Right: If you use formula milks, always be sure to sterilize all your equipment.

Steer clear of fatty as well as fried foods and eat some lean meat, oily fish or pulses every day to keep your iron intake up to replace any that you may have lost in blood during the birth.

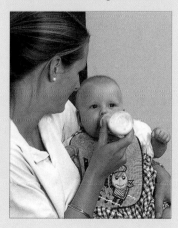

Exercise and relaxation

During pregnancy, exercising is a great way of releasing pent-up tension, increasing your energy levels and paving the way for an easier birth. Try to take a brisk walk outdoors, go for a swim or take some other form of exercise every day – it will make you and your baby feel good. In addition, aerobic exercise can keep blood pressure low and encourage your heart to work more efficiently. When you are trying to conceive, regular exercise can help keep your periods regular, reduce your stress levels, enhance your fertility and improve your sex drive. Exercising also means that you can eat more, so you can increase your vitamin and mineral intake without putting on weight. Don't take up a new energetic sport without taking medical advice.

Exercise During Pregnancy

Gentle exercises such as yoga, Pilates and the Alexander technique are excellent because they focus on posture. Pregnant women are more prone to backache because their centre of gravity is shifted forward and the hormone relaxin softens their ligaments within 4 weeks of conception. Other suitable low-imact exercises include walking, swimming and cycling.

The main rule is to listen to your body and not to overdo the exercise. If you are attending an exercise class, tell your teacher you are pregnant, so that the moves can be adapted to suit you. It is also worth checking out special classes for pregnant women.

Make sure you exercise your upper body too, especially your biceps, in preparation for lifting the baby.

In the first three months after you conceive, you may well feel quite sick and not up to a vigorous workout. Otherwise, most sports are suitable.

From 16-20 weeks on, you should avoid exercising while lying on your back because the weight of the baby can cut off the blood supply in the major vein returning blood from your legs to your heart. This may make you feel dizzy or nauseous.

Avoid abdominal curls from the third month, because the muscles that run down the middle of the tummy may be starting to part. Curls and sit-ups may widen the gap between them, which in turn could mean that it takes longer for your tummy to go down after the birth.

Remember that your heart and lungs are working much harder at this stage, so you will get out of breath more easily and start to feel tired.

From the sixth month, it is best to pace down to a lower level exercise, such as aqua aerobics or walking. During the last three months, high kicks should not be attempted because the pelvis is unstable.

Below: Swimming reduces stress levels, which can enhance fertility, and cushions the joints.

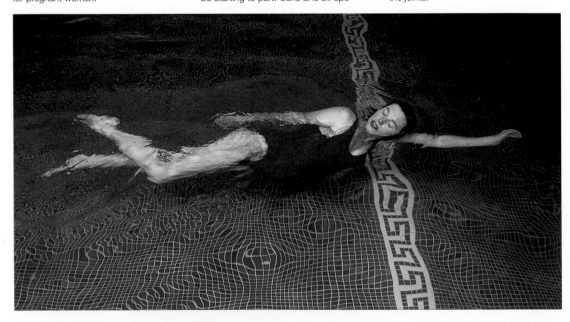

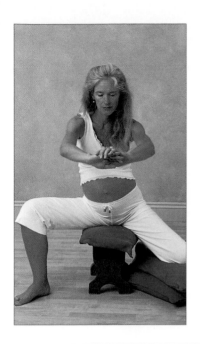

Unwise Exercises

Although it is important to stay fit and healthy during pregnancy, there are some exercises that are unwise because of the changes that are happening to your body. Avoid tennis or high-impact aerobics because these can over-stretch ligaments and cause joint instability.

Although continuing with gentle step classes is acceptable if you are already a regular, do not decide to take up this kind of high impact exercise while you are pregnant. Straining your ligaments can lead to aches and pains after pregnancy and may make you more prone to dislocated bones.

Left: Exercise such as yoga is excellent during pregnancy as it focuses on posture and can help to relieve backache.

Right: Meditation is a good way to relax during pregnancy, as raised stress levels may be harmful to you and your baby.

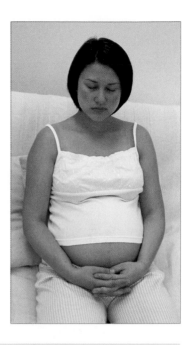

Posture Checks

Exercising the lower abdominals, which are the muscles that feel like a belt around your pelvis, will help the stomach to flatten and return to normal quickly after the birth. This type of exercise should also help to ease the backache caused by carrying extra weight during pregnancy.

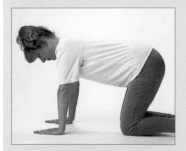

1 Kneel on all fours with your knees shoulder-width apart. Make sure that your hips are aligned above your knees and your neck is in line with your spine.

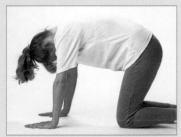

2 As you breathe out, pull the baby up and in towards you, focusing on your abdominal muscles. Hold for 6 seconds, then gently release. Keep your back flat throughout. Do 6–8 repetitions.

This is an exercise that can be adapted to any situation – sitting in the bath, at your desk or waiting in the queue at the supermarket.

Concentrate on pulling the baby up and in towards you, making sure that your tail bone is facing down and your shoulders are back. Keep your head up with your shoulders back and down.

Pelvic Floor Exercises

Start doing these exercises before you become pregnant. The pelvic floor is a sling of muscles running from the tail bone to the pubic bone, which supports the internal organs. Working these muscles daily can help reduce the risk of stress incontinence and can also improve your sex life.

1 In stages, breathe in; breathe out and close your back passage; close the front passage; then, finally, pull up through the middle. Hold for about 6 seconds and then slowly release, with control. You must release fully otherwise you will not feel the full benefit. Repeat about 4–6 times, continuing to breathe throughout.

2 Pull the same muscles up together in one quick action. Hold for about 1 second and slowly release, continuing to breathe throughout. Repeat about 4–6 times.

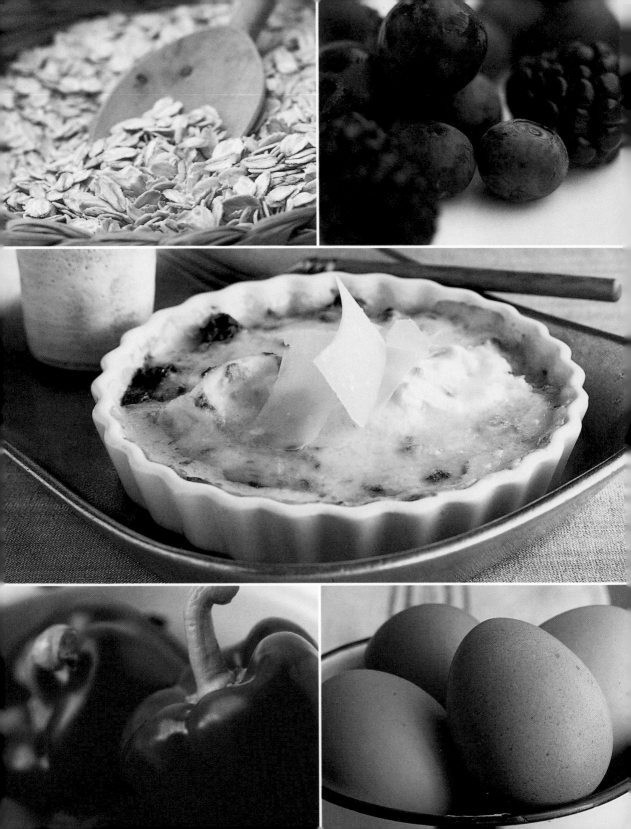

breakfasts and brunches

A well-balanced breakfast based on high carbohydrate foods, such as cereals and grains, will set you up for the day, providing plenty of slow release energy. The recipes in this chapter are packed with the nutrients needed for optimum fertility and a healthy pregnancy: try Luxury Muesli, Apricot and Ginger Compote, or Poached Eggs Florentine. For those who can't face eating early in the morning, there's also a choice of nutritious and refreshing juices and smoothies.

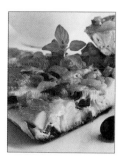 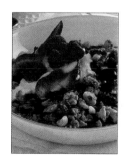 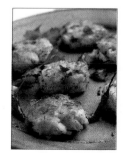

Zingy vegetable juice

An ideal accompaniment to a late Sunday brunch.

Serves 2

1 cooked beetroot (beet) in natural juice, sliced
1 large carrot, sliced
4cm/1½in piece fresh root ginger, finely grated
2 apples, peeled and chopped
150g/5oz/1¼ cups seedless white grapes
300ml/½ pint/1¼ cups fresh orange juice

1 Place the ingredients in a food processor or blender and process until smooth and combined. Pour into glasses and serve immediately.

Nutrition notes	
Per portion:	
Energy	154Kcals/690kJ
Protein	2.3g
Fat	0.4g
saturated fat	0g
Carbohydrate	40.6g
Fibre	3.8g
Calcium	47.2mg
Folate	75.2µg
Vitamin B$_{12}$	0µg
Selenium	2.6µg
Iron	1mg
Zinc	0.3mg

Health benefits

Packed with vitamins, this juice also contains ginger, which is well-known for combating morning sickness.

Cranberry cooler

A great start to the day, or midmorning pick-me-up.

Serves 4

600ml/1 pint/2½ cups cranberry juice
4 eating apples, peeled and sliced
2.5cm/1in piece fresh root ginger, sliced

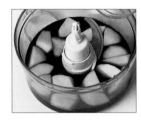

1 Put the cranberry juice and apples into a food processor or blender.

2 Add the ginger to the apples and juice and process until the ingredients are combined and fairly smooth. Serve chilled.

Nutrition notes	
Per portion:	
Energy	108Kcals/451kJ
Protein	0.4g
Fat	0.1g
saturated fat	0g
Carbohydrate	28.5g
Fibre	0g
Calcium	13mg
Folate	1µg
Vitamin B$_{12}$	0µg
Selenium	0µg
Iron	0.1mg
Zinc	0.1mg

Banana smoothie

This breakfast in a glass takes seconds to make.

Serves 2

2 bananas, quartered
225g/8oz strawberries
30ml/2 tbsp oatmeal
600ml/1 pint/2½ cups natural yogurt

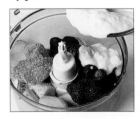

1 Place the bananas, strawberries, oatmeal and natural yogurt in a food processor or blender.

2 Process the ingredients together for a few minutes until thoroughly combined and very creamy. Pour the smoothie into 2 tall glasses and serve at once.

Nutrition notes	
Per portion:	
Energy	317Kcals/1325kJ
Protein	16.6g
Fat	3.7g
saturated fat	1.4g
Carbohydrate	57.8g
Fibre	3.3g
Calcium	508mg
Folate	88.6µg
Vitamin B$_{12}$	0.5µg
Selenium	4.3µg
Iron	1.6mg
Zinc	2.2mg

Citrus shake

Packed with vitamin C, this fruit juice will help you to absorb folates.

Serves 4

1 pineapple
6 oranges, peeled and chopped
1 pink grapefruit, peeled and quartered
juice of 1 lemon

1 Prepare the pineapple: cut the bottom and the spiky top off the fruit. Stand the pineapple upright and cut off the skin, removing all the spikes and as little of the flesh as possible. Lay the pineapple on its side and cut into bitesize chunks.

2 Place all of the fruit and the lemon juice in a food processor or blender and process until combined. Press the juice through a sieve. Serve chilled.

Nutrition notes	
Per portion:	
Energy	117Kcals/493kJ
Protein	2.9g
Fat	0.5g
saturated fat	0g
Carbohydrate	27.3g
Fibre	4.9g
Calcium	120mg
Folate	81.2µg
Vitamin B$_{12}$	0µg
Selenium	3.6µg
Iron	0.5mg
Zinc	0.4mg

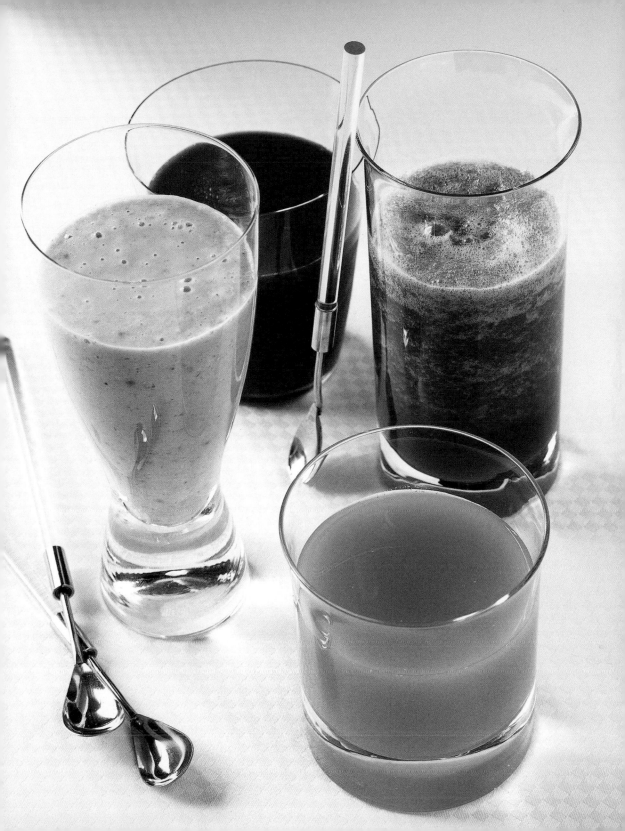

Luxury muesli

This crunchy combination of toasted seeds, grains, nuts and dried fruits provides plenty of slow-release energy to get you through the day. It's delicious served with either milk or a dollop of natural yogurt.

Serves 12

50g/2oz/½ cup sunflower seeds
25g/1oz/¼ cup pumpkin seeds
115g/4oz/1 cup rolled oats
115g/4oz/heaped 1 cup wheat flakes
115g/4oz/heaped 1 cup barley flakes
115g/4oz/⅔ cup raisins
115g/4oz/1 cup chopped hazelnuts, roasted
115g/4oz/½ cup unsulphured dried apricots, chopped
50g/2oz/2 cups dried apple slices, halved
25g/1oz/⅓ cup desiccated (dry unsweetened shredded) coconut

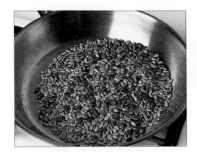

1 Put the sunflower and pumpkin seeds in a small, dry frying pan. Cook over a medium heat for about 3 minutes until golden brown, tossing the seeds regularly to prevent them from burning.

Health benefits

Rolled oats and dried fruit provide an excellent source of soluble fibre that is less harsh on your system than bran.

2 Tip the toasted sunflower and pumpkin seeds into a large bowl and leave to cool. Stir in the rolled oats, wheat and barley flakes, raisins, hazelnuts, dried apricots and apple slices and the coconut. Mix well and leave until completely cold, then store in an airtight container.

Nutrition notes	
Per portion:	
Energy	237Kcals/990kJ
Protein	6g
Fat	11.5g
saturated fat	2g
Carbohydrate	29.6g
Fibre	4.77g
Calcium	40mg
Folate	62.1µg
Vitamin B$_{12}$	0.3µg
Selenium	3.4µg
Iron	5.5mg
Zinc	1.6mg

Granola

Served with milk or yogurt and fresh fruit, this mixture of toasted nuts, seeds, oats and dried fruits will provide a high-calcium, high-fibre start to the day.

Serves 4

115g/4oz/1 cup rolled oats
115g/4oz/1 cup jumbo oats
50g/2oz/ ½ cup sunflower seeds
25g/1oz/2 tbsp sesame seeds
50g/2oz/ ½ cup hazelnuts, roasted
25g/1oz/¼ cup almonds, chopped
60ml/4 tbsp sunflower oil
60ml/4 tbsp clear honey
50g/2oz/⅓ cup raisins
50g/2oz/ ½ cup dried sweetened cranberries

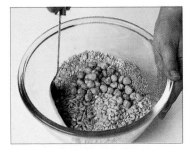

1 Preheat the oven to 140ºC/275ºF/ Gas 1. Mix the oats, seeds and nuts in a bowl. Heat the oil and honey in a large pan until melted, then remove the pan from the heat. Add the oat mixture and stir well. Spread out on baking sheets. Bake for 50 minutes until crisp, stirring occasionally.

2 Mix in the raisins and cranberries. Leave to cool, then store in an airtight container.

Nutrition notes	
Per portion:	
Energy	389Kcals/1625kJ
Protein	9.9g
Fat	23.6g
saturated fat	1.9g
Carbohydrate	38.6g
Fibre	4.9g
Calcium	8.5mg
Folate	35.6µg
Vitamin B$_{12}$	0µg
Selenium	6µg
Iron	3.3mg
Zinc	2.3mg

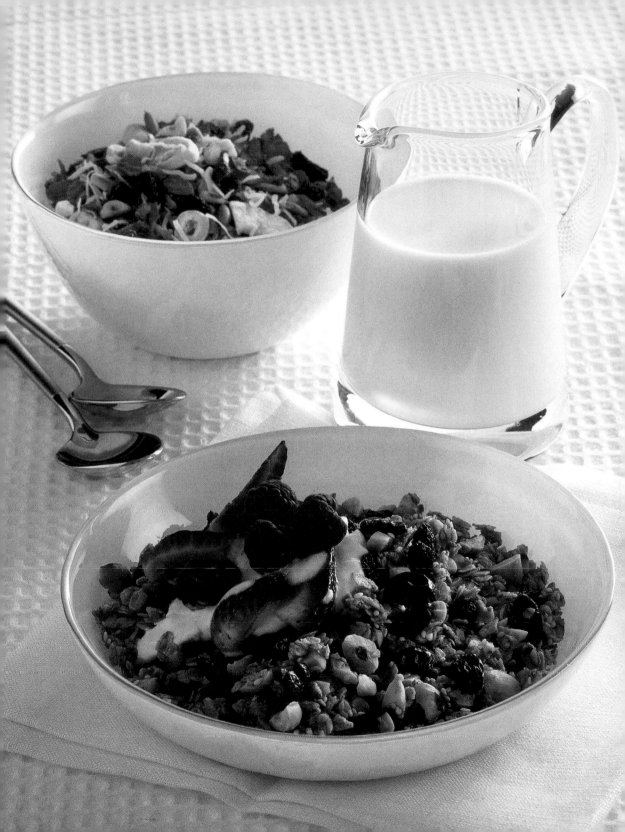

Porridge with date purée and pistachio nuts

Dates are packed with valuable nutrients and fibre, and give a natural sweet flavour to this warming winter breakfast dish.

Serves 4

250g/9oz/scant 2 cups fresh dates
225g/8oz/2 cups rolled oats
475ml/16fl oz/2 cups semi-skimmed (low-fat) milk
pinch of salt
50g/2oz/½ cup shelled, unsalted pistachio nuts, roughly chopped

1 First make the date purée. Halve the dates and remove the stones (pits). Cover the dates with boiling water. Leave to soak for 30 minutes, until softened. Strain the dates, reserving 90ml/6 tbsp of the soaking water.

2 Remove the skin from the dates and place them in a food processor or blender with the reserved water. Process to a smooth purée.

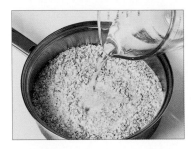

3 Place the oats in a pan with the milk, 300ml/½ pint/1¼ cups water and salt. Bring to the boil, then reduce the heat and simmer for about 4 minutes until cooked and creamy, stirring frequently.

4 Serve the porridge immediately in warm, individual serving bowls, topped with a spoonful of the date purée and sprinkled with the chopped pistachio nuts.

Nutrition notes	
Per portion:	
Energy	399Kcals/1668kJ
Protein	13.1g
Fat	10.7g
saturated fat	1.7g
Carbohydrate	67g
Fibre	5.4g
Calcium	196mg
Folate	60.5µg
Vitamin B$_{12}$	0.5µg
Selenium	3.8µg
Iron	2.7mg
Zinc	2.6mg

Apricot and ginger compote

Fresh ginger adds warmth to this stimulating breakfast dish and complements the flavour of the plump, juicy apricots.

Serves 4

350g/12oz/1½ cups dried unsulphured apricots
4cm/1½in piece fresh root ginger, finely chopped
200g/7oz/scant 1 cup natural (plain) yogurt or low-fat fromage frais, to serve

1 Put the dried apricots in a large heatproof bowl. Pour over enough boiling water to cover, then leave them to soak overnight.

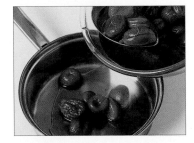

2 Place the apricots and their soaking water in a large heavy-based pan, add the chopped ginger and bring to the boil.

3 Reduce the heat and simmer for 10 minutes until the fruit is soft and plump and the water becomes syrupy.

4 Strain the apricots, reserving the syrup, and discard the chopped ginger. Spoon the warm apricots into individual serving bowls and serve with the reserved syrup and a spoonful of yogurt or fromage frais.

Health benefits

Dried apricots are a good source of iron, which is especially important in the later stages of pregnancy, and they are also an excellent source of soluble fibre.

Nutrition notes	
Per portion:	
Energy	72Kcals/300kJ
Protein	3.3g
Fat	0.5g
saturated fat	0.3g
Carbohydrate	10.1g
Fibre	1.5g
Calcium	10.8mg
Folate	12.8µg
Vitamin B$_{12}$	0.1µg
Selenium	1.4µg
Iron	0.5mg
Zinc	0.4mg

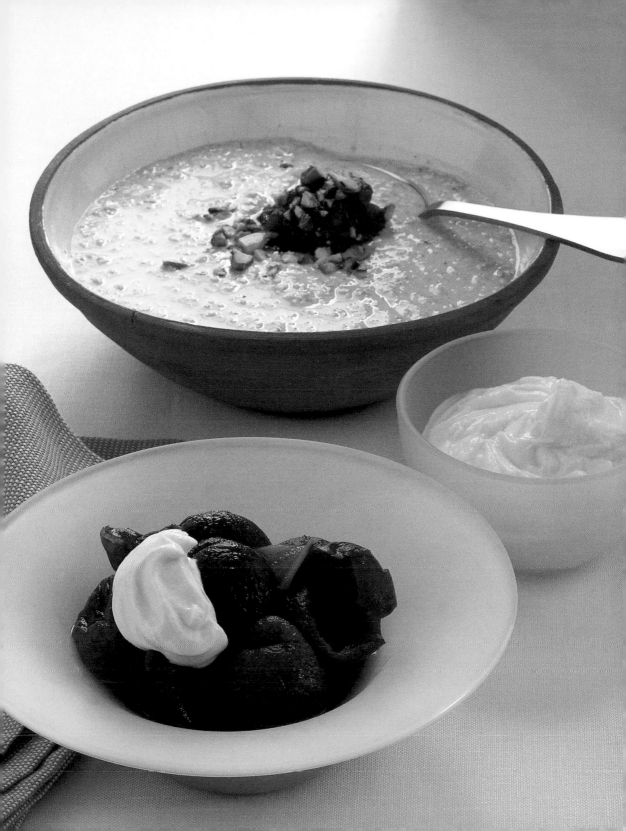

Poached eggs florentine

This hearty brunch dish provides plenty of folates, which are essential before and during the early months of pregnancy.

Serves 4

675g/1½lb spinach
30ml/2 tbsp olive oil
pinch of freshly grated nutmeg
salt and ground black pepper

For the topping
25g/1oz/2 tbsp butter
25g/1oz/¼ cup plain (all-purpose) flour
300ml/½ pint/1¼ cups hot milk
pinch of ground mace
115g/4oz/1 cup Gruyère cheese, grated
4 eggs
15ml/1 tbsp freshly grated Parmesan cheese, plus shaved Parmesan, to serve

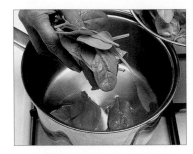

1 Preheat the oven to 200°C/400°F/ Gas 6. Wash and drain the spinach, then place it in a large pan with a little water. Cook for 3–4 minutes until wilted, then drain well. Squeeze out the excess water and then chop finely.

2 Return the chopped spinach to the pan, add the olive oil, nutmeg and seasoning, and heat through. Spoon into four small gratin dishes, making a well in the middle of each.

3 To make the topping, heat the butter in a small pan, add the flour and cook for 1 minute, stirring. Gradually whisk in the hot milk.

4 Cook for 2 minutes, stirring. Remove from the heat and stir in the mace and 75g/3oz/¾ cup of the Gruyère cheese.

5 Break each egg into a cup and slide it into a pan of lightly salted simmering water. Poach for 4–5 minutes until well cooked. Lift out the eggs using a slotted spoon and drain on kitchen paper.

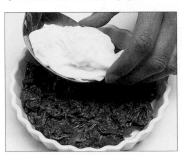

6 Place a poached egg in the middle of each dish and cover with the cheese sauce. Sprinkle the remaining cheeses over the top and bake for about 10 minutes or until just golden. Scatter over a little shaved Parmesan and serve at once.

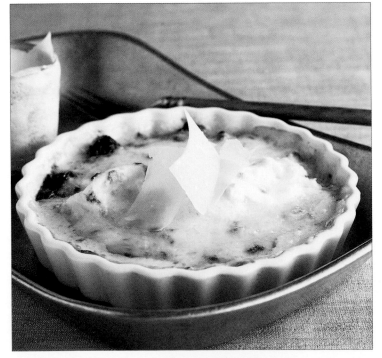

Nutrition notes	
Per portion:	
Energy	283Kcals/1183kJ
Protein	15.1g
Fat	19.8g
saturated fat	7.4g
Carbohydrate	11.3g
Fibre	3.7g
Calcium	461mg
Folate	284.9µg
Vitamin B$_{12}$	1.3µg
Selenium	8.6µg
Iron	4.7mg
Zinc	2.3mg

Soft tacos with spiced scrambled eggs

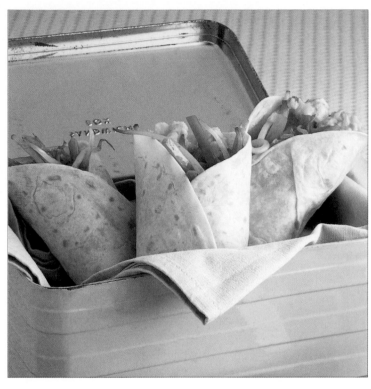

The eggs in these lightly spiced scrambled eggs are a good source of both vitamin B$_{12}$, which is important early in pregnancy, and essential fatty acids, which are important later in pregnancy.

Serves 4

30ml/2 tbsp sunflower oil
50g/2oz beansprouts
50g/2oz carrots, cut into thin sticks
25g/1oz Chinese leaves (cabbage), chopped
15ml/1 tbsp light soy sauce
4 eggs
1 small spring onion (scallion), sliced
5ml/1 tsp Cajun seasoning
30ml/2 tbsp olive oil
4 soft flour tortillas
salt and ground black pepper

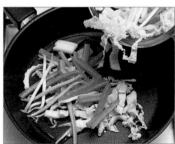

1 Heat the sunflower oil in a frying pan or wok and briefly stir-fry the beansprouts, carrots sticks and Chinese leaves. Add the soy sauce, stir briefly to combine and set aside.

2 In a bowl, beat together the eggs, sliced spring onion, seasoning, salt and ground black pepper, until thoroughly combined.

3 Heat the olive oil in a small pan, add the beaten eggs and cook over a gentle heat, stirring, until firm.

4 Warm the tortillas in the oven or in a microwave, then divide the vegetables and scrambled eggs into four equal portions.

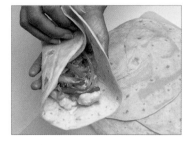

5 Place a portion of the spiced eggs and vegetables in the centre of each warmed tortilla and fold up into cones or parcels. Serve immediately.

Watchpoint

If you are pregnant, be sure to cook the eggs thoroughly as there is a risk that uncooked eggs contain salmonella, which can cause food poisoning.

Nutrition notes

Per portion:

Energy	174Kcals/727kJ
Protein	6.2g
Fat	11.6g
saturated fat	2g
Carbohydrate	12.4g
Fibre	1.2g
Calcium	49mg
Folate	44.3µg
Vitamin B$_{12}$	0.9µg
Selenium	4.7µg
Iron	1.2mg
Zinc	0.6mg

Spanish omelette

This potato and pepper omelette makes a perfect brunch dish both before and during pregnancy. It offers many essential nutrients needed for pre-conception and the developing baby.

Serves 6

30ml/2 tbsp olive oil
1 Spanish onion, chopped
1 small red (bell) pepper, seeded and diced
2 celery sticks, chopped
25g/8oz potatoes, peeled, diced and cooked
400g/14oz can cannellini beans, drained
3 eggs
salt and ground black pepper
sprigs of oregano, to garnish
green salad and olives, to serve

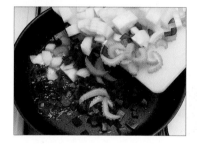

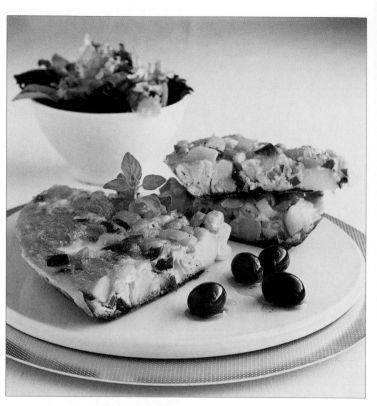

1 Heat the olive oil in a 30cm/12in frying pan or paella pan. Add the onion, red pepper and celery, and cook for 3–5 minutes, stirring occasionally, until the vegetables are softened, but not coloured.

2 Add the potatoes and beans to the pan and heat for several minutes.

3 In a small bowl, beat the eggs with a fork, then season well and pour over the ingredients in the pan. .

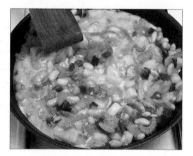

4 Stir the egg mixture to distribute evenly, then allow it to cook over a low heat for about 8 minutes until set. Invert on to a large plate and slide back in to the pan to cook the other side for 2–3 minutes.

5 Cool the omelette slightly, then slide on to a serving plate; cut into wedges. Serve with a green salad and olives. Garnish with oregano.

Health benefits

Eggs offer an excellent supply of vitamin B₁₂ and essential fatty acids, which are important throughout pregnancy. Remember that it is important to cook eggs thoroughly, particularly during pregnancy.

Nutrition notes	
Per portion:	
Energy	244Kcals/1020kJ
Protein	14.9g
Fat	12.6g
saturated fat	2.8g
Carbohydrate	20.1g
Fibre	4.6g
Calcium	70.6mg
Folate	72.3µg
Vitamin B₁₂	2.1µg
Selenium	9.4µg
Iron	2.7mg
Zinc	1.6mg

Spicy crab cakes

Shellfish are a good source of zinc, which is believed to boost fertility, improving sperm count.

Makes about 15

225g/8oz white crab meat (fresh, frozen or canned)
115g/4oz floury potatoes, cooked in salted boiling water, drained and mashed
30ml/2 tbsp fresh herb seasoning
2.5ml/¼ tsp mild mustard
2.5ml/½ tsp ground black pepper
5ml/1 tsp chopped fresh oregano
1 egg, beaten
plain (all-purpose) flour, for dredging
olive oil, for frying
lime wedges, fresh coriander (cilantro) and fresh whole chillies, to garnish

For the tomato dip

15ml/1 tbsp olive oil
½ onion, finely chopped
2 canned plum tomatoes, chopped
1 garlic clove, crushed
150ml/¼ pint/⅔ cup water
5–10ml/1–2 tsp malt vinegar
15ml/1 tbsp chopped fresh coriander (cilantro)
½ fresh hot red chilli, chopped

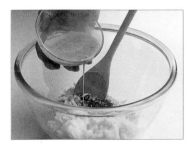

1 Mix together the crab meat, potatoes, seasoning, mustard, pepper, oregano and egg in a large bowl. Chill for 30 minutes.

Watchpoint

Avoid fresh shellfish when pregnant as there is a slight risk of food poisoning.

---

2 Meanwhile, make the tomato dip to accompany the crab cakes. Heat the olive oil in a small pan over a medium heat.

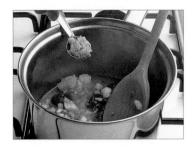

3 Add the onion, tomatoes and garlic to the pan, and sauté for 5 minutes, stirring, until the onion is tender. Add the water, vinegar, coriander and hot chilli. Bring to the boil, then reduce the heat and simmer for about 10 minutes.

4 Transfer the mixture to a food processor or blender and blend to a smooth purée. Pour into a bowl. Keep warm or chill as wished.

5 Using a spoon, shape the crab into rounds and dredge with flour, shaking off the excess. Heat a little oil in a frying pan and fry, a few at a time, for 2–3 minutes on each side. Drain on kitchen paper and keep warm in a low oven while cooking the remainder. Serve with the tomato dip and garnish with lime wedges, coriander sprigs and whole chillies.

Nutrition notes

Per crab cake:

Energy	54Kcals/226kJ
Protein	3.7g
Fat	3.6g
saturated fat	0.6g
Carbohydrate	2.1g
Fibre	0.3g
Calcium	4.7mg
Folate	9.5µg
Vitamin B$_{12}$	0.1µg
Selenium	2.2µg
Iron	0.4mg
Zinc	0.9mg

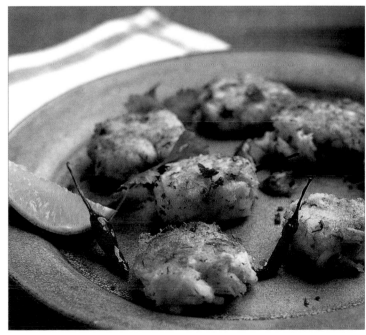

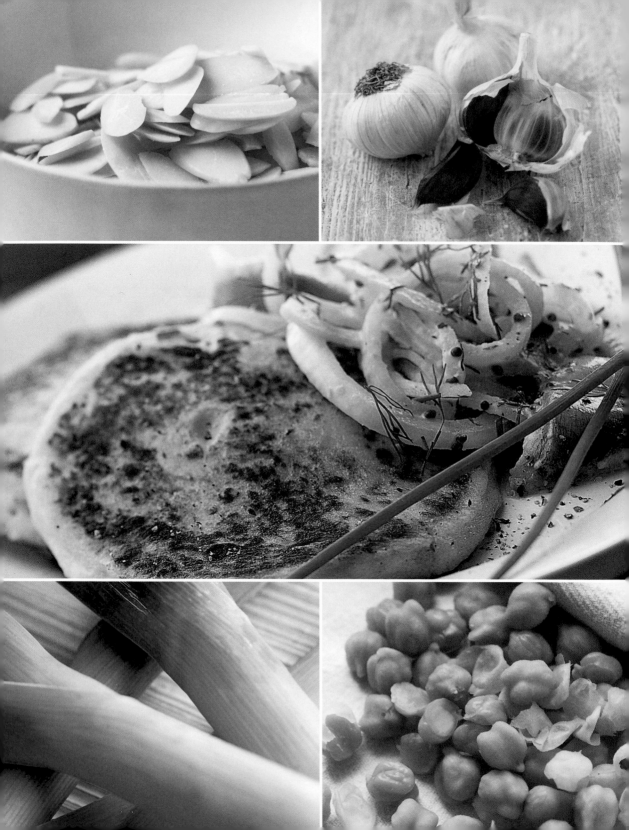

soups and appetizers

When you're pregnant or trying to conceive, soup can make the ideal food. Light soups, such as Miso Broth with Beancurd, are perfect in the first few months when you may not feel much like eating, while hearty, nutritious soups, such as Spinach and Rice Soup, and Pasta, Bean and Vegetable Soup, make a healthy meal in themselves. The fertility-boosing appetizers, such as Sushi and Moules Provençales, are ideal for a romantic dinner.

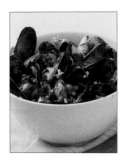 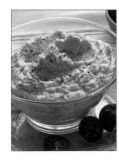 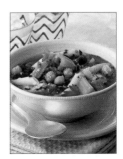

Miso broth with beancurd

Beancurd is a useful source of vitamin E, which is said to promote fertility and boost libido in men. It is also rich in calcium, which is essential for women throughout pregnancy and while breastfeeding.

Serves 4

1 bunch of spring onions (scallions)
   or 5 baby leeks
15g/½oz/½ cup fresh coriander (cilantro)
3 thin slices fresh root ginger
2 star anise
1 small dried red chilli
1.2 litres/2 pints/5 cups dashi stock or
   vegetable stock
225g/8oz pak choi (bok choy) or other
   Asian greens, thickly sliced
200g/7oz firm beancurd (tofu), cubed
60ml/4 tbsp red miso
30–45ml/2–3 tbsp Japanese soy
   sauce (shoyu)
1 fresh red chilli, seeded and shredded (optional)

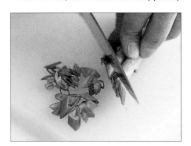

1 Cut off the coarse green tops of the spring onions or baby leeks and place them in a large pan with the coriander stalks, ginger, star anise, dried chilli and dashi or vegetable stock. Heat gently until boiling, then lower the heat and simmer for about 10 minutes.

2 Strain, then return the stock to the pan and reheat. Slice the rest of the onions or leeks finely on the diagonal and add the green portion to the soup with the pak choi or greens and beancurd. Cook for 2 minutes.

3 Mix 45ml/3 tbsp of the miso with a little of the hot soup in a bowl, then stir it into the soup. Add more miso with soy sauce to taste, if needed.

Nutrition notes	
Per portion:	
Energy	55Kcals/230kJ
Protein	5.4g
Fat	2.4g
saturated fat	0.3g
Carbohydrate	3.2g
Fibre	1.6g
Calcium	291mg
Folate	59.1µg
Vitamin B$_{12}$	0µg
Selenium	0.6µg
Iron	1.3mg
Zinc	0.6mg

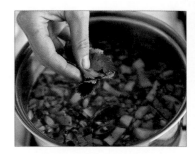

4 Coarsely chop the coriander leaves and stir most of them into the soup with the white part of the spring onions or leeks. Cook for about 1 minute, then ladle the soup into warmed serving bowls. Sprinkle each portion with some of the remaining coriander and the fresh red chilli, if using, and serve at once.

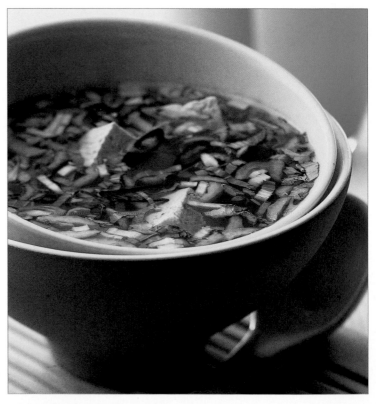

Garlic and almond soup with grapes

This delicately flavoured soup is packed with fertility-boosting vitamin E – great for both men and women before pregnancy.

Serves 6

75g/3oz/¾ cup blanched almonds
50g/2oz/⅔ cup pine nuts
6 large garlic cloves, peeled
175g/6oz crustless day-old bread
1 litre/1¾ pints/4 cups still mineral water, chilled
120ml/4fl oz/½ cup extra virgin olive oil, plus
    extra to serve
15ml/1 tbsp sherry vinegar
30–45ml/2–3 tbsp dry sherry
250g/9oz seedless grapes, peeled
    and halved
salt and ground white pepper
ice cubes and chopped fresh chives,
    to garnish

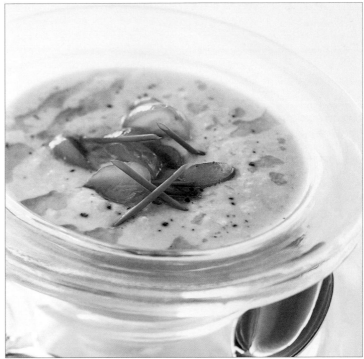

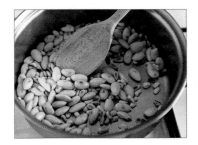

1 Roast the almonds and pine nuts together in a dry pan over a moderate heat until they are very lightly browned. Leave to cool, then grind to a powder.

2 Blanch the garlic in boiling water for 3 minutes. Drain.

3 Put the bread in a shallow bowl, pour over 300ml/½ pint/1¼ cups of the mineral water and leave to soak for 10 minutes, then squeeze dry. Mix the garlic, bread, nuts and 5ml/1 tsp salt in a food processor or blender and pulse the mixture until it forms a smooth paste.

4 Gradually blend in the olive oil and sherry vinegar, followed by sufficient water to make a smooth soup with a creamy consistency.

5 Stir in 30ml/2 tbsp of the sherry. Adjust the seasoning, then add more sherry to taste. Chill for at least 3 hours, then adjust the seasoning again and stir in a little more chilled water if the soup has thickened. Reserve a few of the grapes for the garnish and stir the remainder into the chilled soup.

6 Ladle the soup into bowls (glass bowls look particularly good) and garnish with ice cubes, the reserved grapes and chopped fresh chives. Serve with additional extra virgin olive oil to drizzle over the soup.

Nutrition notes	
Per portion:	
Energy	404Kcals/1689kJ
Protein	6.9g
Fat	31.7g
saturated fat	3.7g
Carbohydrate	24.3g
Fibre	2g
Calcium	73.6mg
Folate	13.3µg
Vitamin B$_{12}$	0µg
Selenium	10.9µg
Iron	1.6mg
Zinc	1.2mg

Health benefits

Almonds are an excellent source of fertility-boosting vitamin E. They are also a good source of calcium, which is essential for pregnant women as it helps to avoid loss of calcium from the bones.

Spinach and rice soup

This tasty, wholesome soup is great for pre-conception and the first few months of pregnancy.

Serves 4

675g/1½ lb fresh spinach leaves, washed
45ml/3 tbsp extra virgin olive oil
1 small onion, finely chopped
2 garlic cloves, finely chopped
1 small fresh red chilli, seeded and finely chopped
225g/8oz/generous 1 cup risotto rice
1.2 litres/2 pints/5 cups vegetable stock
salt and ground black pepper
Parmesan cheese shavings, to serve

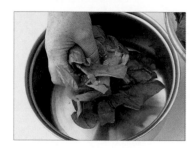

1 Place the spinach in a large pan with just the water that clings to its leaves after washing. Add a large pinch of salt. Heat gently until the spinach has wilted, then remove from the heat and drain, reserving any liquid.

2 Either chop the spinach finely using a large kitchen knife or place in a food processor and process the leaves to a fairly coarse purée.

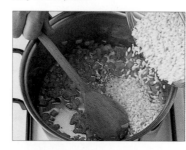

3 Heat the oil in a large pan and gently cook the onion, garlic and chilli for 4–5 minutes until the onion is softened. Stir in the rice until well coated, then pour in the stock and reserved spinach liquid. Bring to the boil, then lower the heat and simmer for 10 minutes.

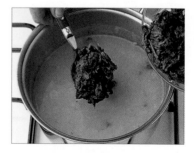

4 Add the spinach, with salt and pepper to taste. Cook for 5–7 minutes, until the rice is tender. Check the seasoning. Serve in heated bowls, topped with the shavings of cheese.

Health benefits

Leafy green vegetables like spinach are rich in folates, which can help to protect your baby from neural tube defects.

Nutrition notes	
Per portion:	
Energy	323Kcals/1350kJ
Protein	9.6g
Fat	10.5g
saturated fat	1.4g
Carbohydrate	46g
Fibre	3.7g
Calcium	299mg
Folate	255µg
Vitamin B_{12}	0µg
Selenium	1.8µg
Iron	4.3mg
Zinc	2.5mg

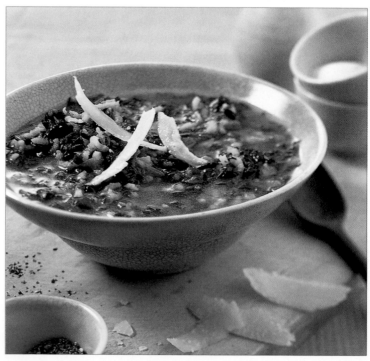

Pasta, bean and vegetable soup

This hearty soup is very rich in selenium and contains iron. Both nutrients are important before conception, during pregnancy and while breastfeeding.

Serves 4–6

75g/3oz/scant ½ cup brown lentils
15g/½ oz/¼ cup dried porcini mushrooms
60ml/4 tbsp extra virgin olive oil
1 carrot, diced
1 celery stick, diced
1 onion, finely chopped
1 garlic clove, finely chopped
a little chopped fresh flat leaf parsley
a good pinch of crushed red
    chillies (optional)
1.5 litres/2½ pints/6¼ cups well-flavoured
    vegetable stock
150g/5oz/scant 1 cup each canned red kidney
    beans, cannellini beans and chickpeas, rinsed
    and drained
115g/4oz/1 cup small dried pasta shapes, such
    as rigatoni, penne or penne rigate
salt and ground black pepper
chopped flat leaf parsley, to garnish
freshly grated Pecorino cheese, to serve

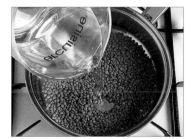

1 Put the lentils in a medium pan and add 475ml/16fl oz/2 cups water. Bring to the boil over a high heat. Lower the heat to a gentle simmer and cook, stirring occasionally, for 15–20 minutes or until the lentils are just tender.

2 Meanwhile, soak the dried mushrooms in 175ml/6fl oz/¾ cup warm water for 15–20 minutes.

3 Tip the lentils into a colander to drain, then rinse under the cold tap. Drain the soaked mushrooms, reserving the soaking liquid. Finely chop the mushrooms and set aside.

4 Heat the oil in a large pan and add the carrot, celery, onion, garlic, parsley and crushed chillies, if using. Cook over a low heat, stirring constantly, for 5–7 minutes.

5 Add the stock, mushrooms and their soaking liquid to the pan. Bring to the boil, then add the beans, chickpeas and lentils and season. Cover, and simmer for about 20 minutes.

Cook's tip

You can freeze the soup at the end of Step 5. Thaw, then add the pasta when reheating.

---

6 Add the pasta and bring the soup back to the boil, stirring. Simmer, stirring frequently, for 7–8 minutes or until the pasta is cooked. Season, then serve hot in soup bowls, with grated Pecorino and chopped parsley.

Nutrition notes	
Per portion:	
Energy	207Kcals/865kJ
Protein	7.8g
Fat	8.3g
saturated fat	1.2g
Carbohydrate	27g
Fibre	4.1g
Calcium	41.1mg
Folate	24.3µg
Vitamin B$_{12}$	0µg
Selenium	20.8µg
Iron	2.5mg
Zinc	1.11mg

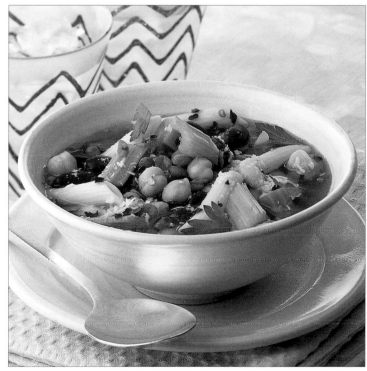

Chicken and leek soup with prunes

This flavourful, high fibre soup provides plenty of iron, protein and slow-release energy.

Serves 6

1 chicken, about 2kg/4½lb
900g/2lb leeks
1 fresh bay leaf
a few each fresh parsley stalks and
    thyme sprigs
1 large carrot, thickly sliced
2.5 litres/4 pints/10 cups chicken or
    beef stock
115g/4oz/generous ½ cup pearl barley
400g/14oz/1¾ cups ready-to-eat prunes
salt and ground black pepper
chopped fresh parsley, to garnish

1 Cut the breasts off the chicken and set aside. Place the remaining chicken carcass in a large pan. Cut half the leeks into 5cm/2in lengths and add them to the pan. Tie the herbs into a bouquet garni and add to the pan with the carrot and the stock.

2 Bring the mixture to the boil, then reduce the heat and cover. Simmer gently for 1 hour. Skim off any scum when the water first boils and again from time to time during simmering.

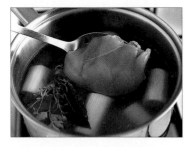

3 Add the chicken breasts and cook for another 30 minutes, until they are just cooked. Leave until cool enough to handle, then strain the stock. Reserve the chicken breasts and meat from the carcass. Discard the skin, bones, cooked vegetables and herbs.

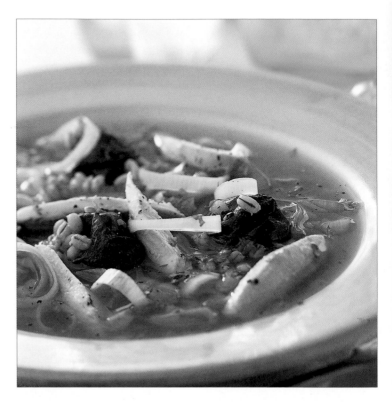

4 Meanwhile, rinse the pearl barley thoroughly in a sieve under cold running water, then cook it in a large pan of boiling water for about 10 minutes. Drain, rinse well again and drain thoroughly.

5 Skim as much fat as you can from the stock, then return it to the pan. Add the pearl barley. Bring to the boil over a medium heat, then lower the heat and cook very gently for 15–20 minutes, until the barley is just cooked and tender. Season the soup with 5ml/1 tsp salt and plenty of black pepper to taste.

6 Add the prunes. Thinly slice the remaining leeks and add them to the pan. Bring to the boil, then lower the heat and simmer for 10 minutes or until the leeks are just cooked.

7 Slice the chicken breasts and add them to the soup with the remaining chicken meat, sliced or cut into neat pieces. Reheat if necessary. Serve sprinkled with chopped parsley.

Nutrition notes	
Per portion:	
Energy	674Kcals/2817kJ
Protein	46.3g
Fat	35.7g
saturated fat	10.1g
Carbohydrate	44.1g
Fibre	7.4g
Calcium	82.5mg
Folate	104µg
Vitamin B_{12}	0µg
Selenium	30.5µg
Iron	5mg
Zinc	3.3mg

Hummus

This spicy chickpea dip makes a great appetizer or snack before and during pregnancy and while breastfeeding. It provides valuable folates, iron and fibre.

Serves 4-6

150g/5oz/¾ cup dried chickpeas
juice of 2 lemons
2 garlic cloves, sliced
30ml/2 tbsp olive oil
pinch of cayenne pepper
150ml/¼ pint/⅔ cup tahini paste
salt and ground black pepper
extra olive oil and cayenne pepper, for
   sprinkling
fresh flat leaf parsley and cherry tomatoes,
   to garnish

1 Put the chickpeas in a bowl with plenty of cold water and leave to soak overnight.

2 Drain the chickpeas and put them in a large pan. Add fresh cold water to cover. Bring to the boil and boil rapidly for 10 minutes, then reduce the heat and simmer gently for about 1 hour until soft. Drain.

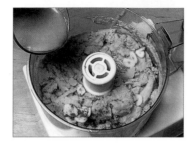

3 Process the chickpeas in a food processor to a smooth paste. Add the lemon juice, garlic, olive oil, cayenne pepper and tahini and blend again until creamy, scraping the mixture down from the sides of the bowl.

4 Season the hummus with salt and ground black pepper and transfer to a serving dish. Sprinkle with oil and cayenne pepper and garnish with parsley sprigs. Serve with cherry tomatoes. Hummus is also good with raw vegetable crudités.

Nutrition notes	
Per portion:	
Energy	163Kcals/681kJ
Protein	6.8g
Fat	9.8g
saturated fat	1.4g
Carbohydrate	12.5g
Fibre	3.3g
Calcium	96.7mg
Folate	53.5µg
Vitamin B$_{12}$	0µg
Selenium	0.5µg
Iron	2.3mg
Zinc	1.2mg

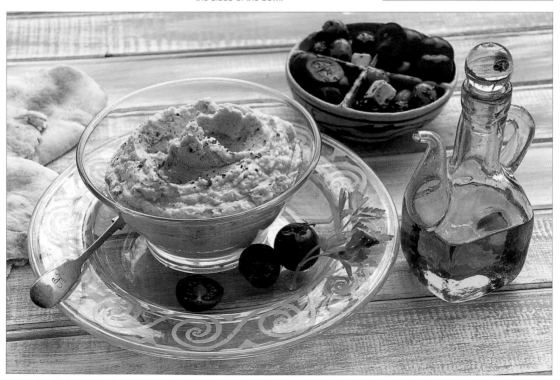

Yogurt and cucumber dip

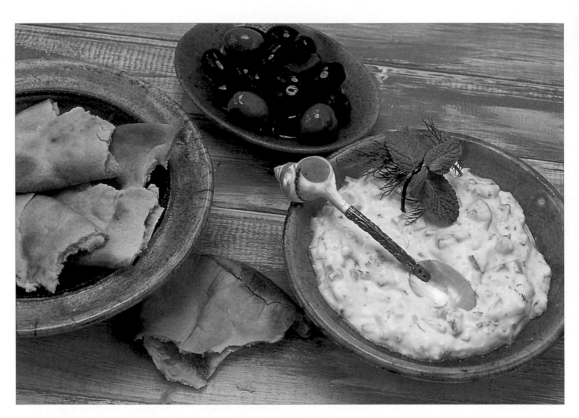

Yogurt is an excellent source of calcium, which is an important nutrient for pregnant women and breastfeeding mothers, and will help to prevent the loss of this mineral from bones. Yogurt also contains B vitamins, which are needed before conception.

Serves 6

1 small cucumber
300ml/½ pint/1¼ cups thick natural (plain) yogurt
3 garlic cloves, crushed
30ml/2 tbsp chopped fresh mint
30ml/2 tbsp chopped fresh dill or parsley
salt and ground black pepper
mint or parsley and dill, to garnish
olive oil, olives and pitta bread, to serve

1 Finely chop the cucumber and layer in a colander with plenty of salt. Leave for 30 minutes. Wash the cucumber well and drain thoroughly.

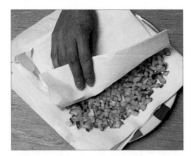

2 Lay a sheet of kitchen paper on a plate and spread out the chopped cucumber on top. Cover with more kitchen paper and blot the cucumber dry.

3 Mix the yogurt, garlic and herbs and season well. Stir in the cucumber. Garnish with herbs, drizzle olive oil over and serve with olives and pitta bread.

Nutrition notes	
Per portion:	
Energy	30Kcals/125kJ
Protein	2.6g
Fat	0.4g
saturated fat	0.3g
Carbohydrate	4g
Fibre	0.1g
Calcium	98mg
Folate	10µg
Vitamin B$_{12}$	0.1µg
Selenium	0.5µg
Iron	0.1mg
Zinc	0.1mg

Sushi

Seaweed is a good source of vitamin B$_{12}$, which is needed for pre-conception.

Makes 12 rolls or 72 slices

400g/14oz/2 cups sushi rice, soaked for 20
    minutes in water to cover
55ml/3½ tbsp rice vinegar
15ml/1 tbsp granulated sugar
2.5ml/½ tsp salt
6 sheets nori seaweed
200g/7oz tuna, in one piece
200g/7oz salmon, in one piece
wasabi paste
½ cucumber, quartered lengthways
    and seeded
pickled ginger, to garnish (optional)
Japanese soy sauce (shoyu), to serve

1 Drain the rice, then put it in a pan with 550ml/18fl oz/2½ cups water. Bring to the boil, then lower the heat, cover and simmer for 20 minutes, or until the liquid has been absorbed. Meanwhile, heat the vinegar, sugar and salt, stir well and cool. Add to the rice, then remove the pan from the heat and allow to stand, covered, for about 20 minutes.

2 Cut the nori sheets in half lengthways. Cut the tuna, salmon and cucumber into four long sticks, each about the same length as the nori, and 1cm/½in square.

3 Place a sheet of nori, shiny side down, on a bamboo mat. Divide the cooked rice into 12 equal portions. Spread one portion of rice over the nori sheet, leaving 1cm/½in clear at each end.

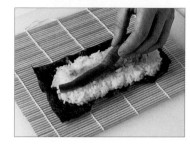

4 Spread a small amount of wasabi paste in a horizontal line along the middle of the rice. Lay one or two sticks of tuna on top, making sure the fish reaches the end of the rice.

5 Holding the mat and the edge of the nori sheet, roll up the nori and rice into a narrow cylinder with the tuna in the middle. Use the mat as a guide – do not roll it into the food. Roll the rice tightly so that it sticks together and encloses the filling firmly.

6 Carefully roll the sushi off the mat. Make 11 more rolls in the same way, four for each filling, but do not use wasabi with the cucumber. Use a wet knife to cut each roll into six slices and stand them on a platter. Garnish with pickled ginger, if liked, and serve with the soy sauce.

Watchpoint

It is best to avoid raw fish when pregnant so try making this recipe with strips of cooked salmon and tuna instead.

Nutrition notes	
Per portion:	
Energy	31Kcals/129kJ
Protein	1.8g
Fat	0.6g
saturated fat	0.1g
Carbohydrate	4.8g
Fibre	0.3g
Calcium	6.9mg
Folate	2µg
Vitamin B$_{12}$	0.4µg
Selenium	2.8µg
Iron	0.2mg
Zinc	0.2mg

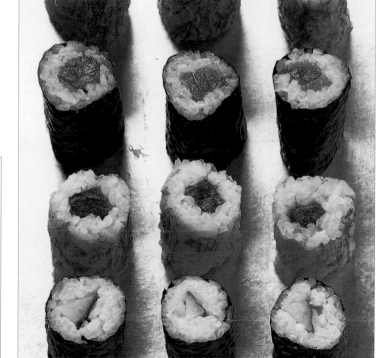

Potato pancakes with pickled herring

Herring are a great source of omega-3 fatty acids, which are important in the second and third trimesters, and calcium, which is an essential nutrient for breastfeeding mothers.

Serves 6

2 peeled potatoes, about 275g/10oz
2 eggs, beaten
150ml/¼ pint/⅔ cup milk
40g/1½oz/6 tbsp plain (all-purpose) flour
30ml/2 tbsp chopped fresh chives
olive oil, for greasing
salt and ground black pepper
fresh dill sprigs and fresh chives,
    to garnish

For the topping
2 small onions, thinly sliced into rings
60ml/4 tbsp crème fraîche
5ml/1 tsp wholegrain mustard
15ml/1 tbsp chopped fresh dill
6 pickled herring fillets

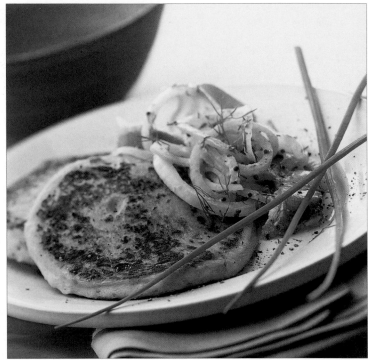

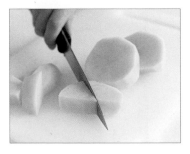

1 Cut the potatoes into chunks and cook them in boiling salted water for about 15 minutes or until tender. Drain well, then return the potatoes to the pan and mash or press through a wide-meshed sieve (strainer) to form a smooth purée.

2 Meanwhile, prepare the topping. Place the onion rings in a large bowl and cover with boiling water. Set aside for 2–3 minutes, then drain thoroughly and dry on kitchen paper.

3 Mix the onion rings with the crème fraîche, mustard and chopped dill. Season to taste. Using a sharp knife, cut the pickled herring fillets into 12–18 pieces. Set them aside.

4 Put the potato purée in a bowl and whisk in the eggs, milk and flour to make a batter. Season with salt and pepper and whisk in the chopped chives.

5 Heat a non-stick frying pan over a medium heat and grease it with a little oil. Spoon about 30ml/2 tbsp of batter into the pan to make a pancake, measuring about 7.5cm/3in across. Cook for 3 minutes, until the underside is set and golden brown.

6 Turn the pancake over and cook the other side for 3–4 minutes, until golden brown. Transfer to a plate and keep warm while you make the remaining pancakes.

7 Place two pancakes on each of six warmed plates and distribute the herring and onion mixture equally among them. Garnish with dill sprigs and chives. Season with black pepper and serve immediately.

Nutrition notes	
Per portion:	
Energy	270Kcals/1129kJ
Protein	16.3g
Fat	14.9g
saturated fat	3g
Carbohydrate	17.9g
Fibre	0.7g
Calcium	21.5mg
Folate	19.4µg
Vitamin B$_{12}$	0µg
Selenium	0.6µg
Iron	0.9mg
Zinc	0.5mg

Moules provençal

Mussels, like all shellfish, are an excellent source of fertility-boosting zinc. This valuable nutrient is needed for a good sperm count.

Serves 4

30ml/2 tbsp olive oil
200g/7oz rindless unsmoked streaky (fatty) bacon, chopped
1 onion, finely chopped
3 garlic cloves, finely chopped
1 bay leaf
15ml/1 tbsp chopped fresh mixed Provençal herbs, such as thyme, marjoram, basil, oregano and savory
15–30ml/1–2 tbsp sun-dried tomatoes in oil, drained and chopped
4 large, very ripe tomatoes, peeled, seeded and chopped
50g/2oz/½ cup pitted black olives, chopped
105ml/7 tbsp dry white wine
2.25kg/5lb mussels, scrubbed and bearded, discard any that are open
salt and ground black pepper
60ml/4 tbsp coarsely chopped fresh parsley, to garnish
French bread, cut into chunks, to serve

1 Heat the oil in a large pan. Fry the bacon until golden and crisp. Remove with a slotted spoon; set aside. Add the onion and garlic to the pan and cook, stirring, until softened.

2 Add the herbs, with both types of tomatoes to the pan. Fry gently for 5 minutes, stirring. Stir in the olives and season with salt and pepper.

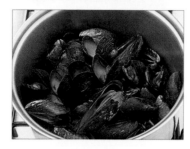

3 Put the white wine and mussels in another pan. Cover and cook over a high heat for 5 minutes, shaking the pan frequently, until the mussels open. Discard any that remain closed.

4 Strain the cooking liquid into the pan containing the tomato sauce and boil until reduced by about one-third. Add the cooked mussels and stir with a wooden spoon to coat them thoroughly with the sauce. Take out the bay leaf and discard.

5 Divide the mussels and sauce among four heated dishes. Scatter over the fried bacon and chopped parsley and serve piping hot, with French bread for mopping up the delectable juices.

Watchpoint

Although mussels contain nutrients that are excellent for pre-conception, they are a common cause of food poisoning so should be avoided during pregnancy.

Nutrition notes

Per portion:

Energy	525Kcals/2194kJ
Protein	47.6g
Fat	21.6g
saturated fat	7g
Carbohydrate	10g
Fibre	2.4g
Calcium	153mg
Folate	149µg
Vitamin B$_{12}$	59.8µg
Selenium	163µg
Iron	19.6mg
Zinc	8.9mg

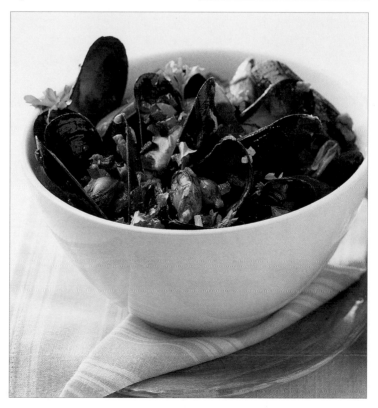

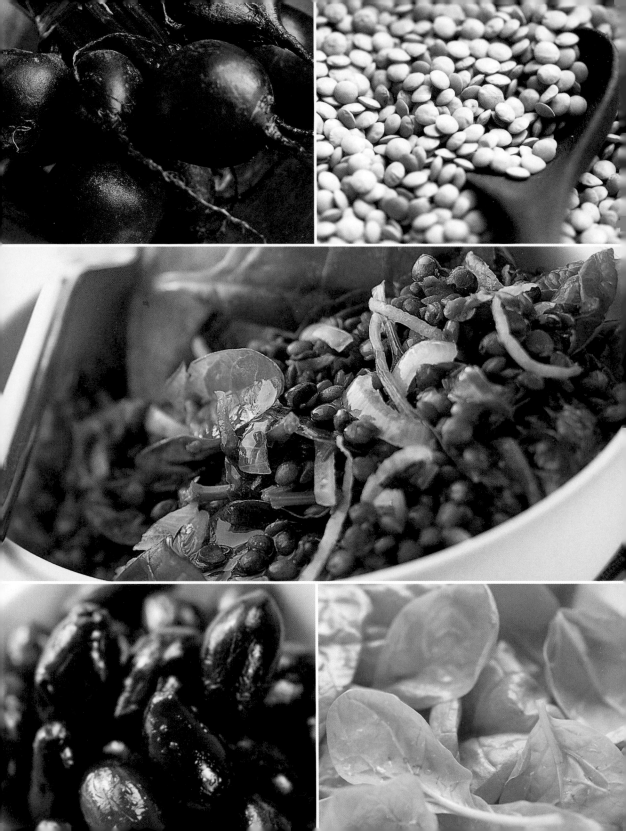

salads and light meals

These healthy and quick-to-cook meals have been designed
to carry you through pre-conception, pregnancy and breastfeeding.
Each dish is packed with nutritious ingredients, such as beans,
nuts, eggs and fish, which are vital for a healthy baby. Try
Fruit and Vegetable Salad with Peanut Sauce, or Salad Niçoise,
or choose a hot meal such as Tagliatelle with Broccoli and
Spinach. These little dishes are also ideal to eat later in
pregnancy, when big meals may cause indigestion.

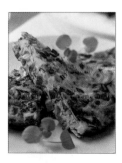
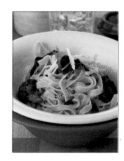
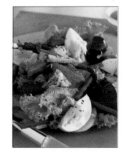

Sardine and black olive salad

Sardines, eaten with their bones, are a good source of calcium and also contain essential fatty acids, protein, iron and zinc. This wealth of nutrients makes this dish perfect, any time from pre-conception through to breastfeeding.

Serves 6

8 large firm ripe tomatoes
1 large red onion
60ml/4 tbsp wine vinegar
90ml/6 tbsp good olive oil
18–24 small sardines, cooked
75g/3oz/¾ cup stoned (pitted) black olives, well
    drained
salt and ground black pepper
45ml/3 tbsp chopped fresh parsley,
    to garnish

1 Cut the tomatoes into 5mm/¼in slices. Slice the onion thinly.

2 Divide the tomatoes among six plates, overlapping the slices, then top with the red onion.

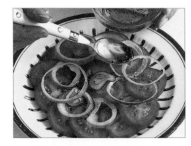

3 Mix together the wine vinegar, olive oil and seasoning and spoon over the tomatoes.

4 Top each portion with 3–4 sardines and several black olives. Sprinkle the chopped parsley over the top and serve at once.

Nutrition notes	
Per portion:	
Energy	148Kcals/618kJ
Protein	1.6g
Fat	12.8g
saturated fat	1.9g
Carbohydrate	7.3g
Fibre	2.3g
Calcium	26.9mg
Folate	29.4µg
Vitamin B$_{12}$	0µg
Selenium	0.4µg
Iron	0.9mg
Zinc	0.2mg

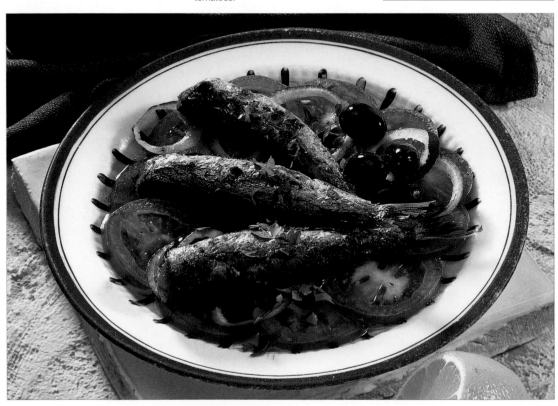

Beetroot and red onion salad

This light, refreshing and colourful salad contains walnuts, which are high in vitamin E, folates and omega-3 fatty acids. These nutrients are all essential both before conception and during pregnancy.

Serves 6

500g/1¼lb small beetroot (beet)
75ml/5 tbsp water
60ml/4 tbsp olive oil
90g/3½oz/scant 1 cup walnut halves
5ml/1 tsp caster (superfine) sugar, plus a little extra for the dressing
30ml/2 tbsp walnut oil
15ml/1 tbsp sherry vinegar or balsamic vinegar
5ml/1 tsp soy sauce
5ml/1 tsp grated orange rind
2.5ml/½ tsp ground roasted coriander seeds
5–10ml/1–2 tsp orange juice
1 red onion, halved and very thinly sliced, separated
15–30ml/1–2 tbsp chopped fresh fennel
75g/3oz watercress or mizuna leaves
handful of baby red chard or beetroot (beet) leaves (optional)
salt and ground black pepper

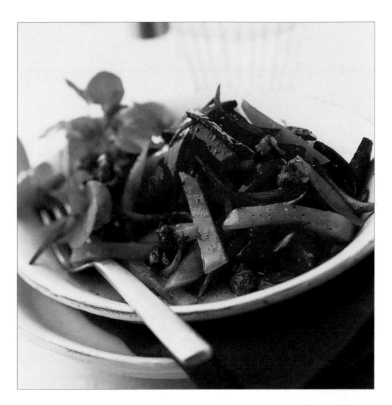

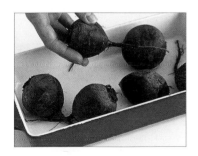

1 Preheat the oven to 180°C/350°F/ Gas 4. Place the beetroot in an ovenproof dish just large enough to hold them in a single layer and add the water. Cover tightly and cook in the oven for 1–1½ hours, or until they are just tender.

2 Cool, then peel the beetroot and cut them into strips or slice them. Toss with 15ml/1 tbsp of the olive oil. Transfer to a bowl and set aside.

3 Heat about 15ml/1 tbsp of the remaining olive oil in a small frying pan and cook the walnuts until they begin to brown. Add the sugar and cook, stirring, until the nuts begin to caramelize. Season with 2.5ml/½ tsp salt and lots of pepper, then turn the nuts out on to a plate and leave to cool.

4 In a jug (pitcher) or bowl, whisk together the remaining olive oil, the walnut oil, sherry or balsamic vinegar, soy sauce, orange rind and ground roasted coriander seeds to make the dressing. Season with salt and pepper to taste and add a pinch of caster sugar. Whisk in orange juice to taste.

5 Toss the onion slices with the beetroot strips and dressing, then add the fennel, watercress or mizuna and red chard or beetroot leaves. Toss again and serve, sprinkled with the caramelized nuts.

Nutrition notes	
Per portion:	
Energy	238Kcals/995kJ
Protein	4.1g
Fat	21.5g
saturated fat	2.3g
Carbohydrate	7.7g
Fibre	2.4g
Calcium	54.5mg
Folate	136µg
Vitamin B$_{12}$	0µg
Selenium	2.9µg
Iron	1.6mg
Zinc	0.9mg

Brown bean salad

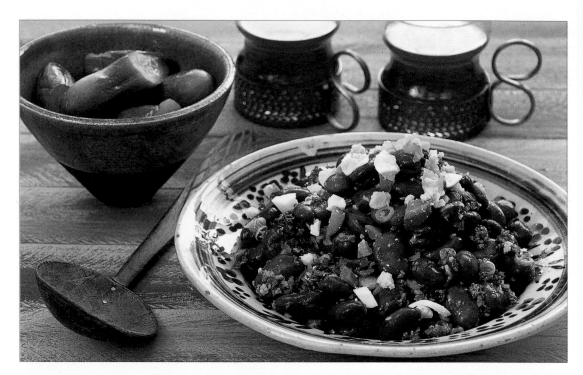

This high-fibre egg and bean salad is full of nutrients, such as folates and iron, and is good to eat from pre-conception right through to the later stages of pregnancy.

Serves 6

350g/12oz/1½ cups dried brown beans (ful medames)
3 fresh thyme sprigs
2 bay leaves
1 onion, halved
4 garlic cloves, crushed
7.5ml/1½ tsp cumin seeds, crushed
3 spring onions (scallions), finely chopped
90ml/6 tbsp chopped fresh parsley
20ml/4 tsp lemon juice
90ml/6 tbsp olive oil
3 hard-boiled (hard-cooked) eggs, roughly chopped
1 pickled cucumber, roughly chopped
salt and ground black pepper

Nutrition notes	
Per portion:	
Energy	305Kcals/1275kJ
Protein	15.1g
Fat	14.0g
saturated fat	2.4g
Carbohydrate	31.6g
Fibre	6.9g
Calcium	76.8mg
Folate	15.1µg
Vitamin B$_{12}$	0.2µg
Selenium	4.2µg
Iron	3.1mg
Zinc	3.3mg

1 Put the beans in a bowl with plenty of cold water and leave to soak overnight. Drain, rinse under cold water and drain again. Transfer to a large pan and cover with fresh water. Bring to the boil and boil rapidly for 10 minutes.

2 Reduce the heat, add the sprigs of thyme, bay leaves and onion, then simmer very gently for about 1 hour until the beans are tender. Drain and discard the herbs and onion halves.

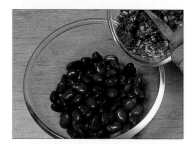

3 Mix together the garlic, cumin, spring onions, parsley, lemon juice and oil, and add a little salt and pepper. Pour over the beans and toss together.

4 Gently stir in the chopped eggs and cucumber and serve at once.

Lentil and spinach salad

This wonderful salad is good anytime, but is particularly beneficial for pre-conception and early pregnancy because of the high levels of folates found in both lentils and spinach.

Serves 6

225g/8oz/1 cup Puy lentils
1 fresh bay leaf
1 celery stick
fresh thyme sprig
30ml/2 tbsp olive oil
1 onion or 3–4 shallots, finely chopped
10ml/2 tsp crushed toasted cumin seeds
400g/14oz young spinach
salt and ground black pepper
30–45ml/2–3 tbsp chopped fresh parsley, plus a
    few extra sprigs

For the dressing

75ml/5 tbsp extra virgin olive oil
5ml/1 tsp Dijon mustard
about 15ml/1 tbsp red wine vinegar
1 small garlic clove, finely chopped
2.5ml/½ tsp finely grated lemon rind

1 Rinse the lentils and place them in a large pan. Add plenty of water to cover. Tie the bay leaf, celery and thyme into a bundle and add to the pan, then bring to the boil. Reduce the heat so that the water boils steadily. Cook the lentils for 30–45 minutes, until just tender. Do not add salt.

2 Meanwhile, make the dressing by whisking all the ingredients together. Season well.

3 Thoroughly drain the lentils and tip them into a large bowl. Add most of the dressing and toss well, then set the lentils aside, stirring occasionally.

4 Heat the oil in a deep frying pan and cook the onion or shallots over a low heat for about 4–5 minutes, until they are beginning to soften. Add the cumin and cook for 1 minute.

5 Add the spinach to the pan and season to taste. Cover and cook for about 2 minutes. Stir, then cook again briefly until the spinach has wilted.

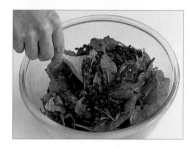

6 Stir the spinach into the lentils and leave to cool. Chill until ready to serve, then bring back to room temperature if necessary. Stir in the remaining dressing and the chopped parsley and adjust the seasoning if necessary.

7 Taste the salad and add more red wine vinegar, if needed. Serve in warmed individual bowls, with slices of toasted bread or chunks of rough wholegrain bread, if you like.

Nutrition notes	
Per portion:	
Energy	252Kcals/1053kJ
Protein	11.3g
Fat	14.1g
saturated fat	1.9g
Carbohydrate	21.4g
Fibre	5.1g
Calcium	148mg
Folate	146µg
Vitamin B$_{12}$	0µg
Selenium	40.4µg
Iron	5.7mg
Zinc	1.9mg

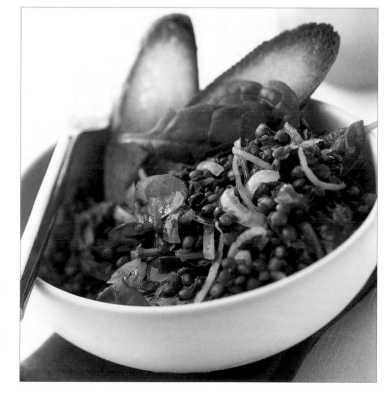

Fruit and vegetable salad with peanut sauce

Perfect for pre-conception and early pregnancy, this dish is rich in folates and vitamin C, to help its absorption. Peanuts are also rich in zinc, magnesium and iron.

Serves 6

½ cucumber
2 pears (not too ripe)
1–2 eating apples
juice of ½ lemon
mixed salad leaves
6 small tomatoes, cut in wedges
3 slices fresh pineapple, cored and cut in wedges
3 hard-boiled (hard-cooked) eggs, quartered
175g/6oz egg noodles, cooked, cooled and chopped

For the peanut sauce

2–4 fresh red chillies, seeded and ground, or 15ml/1 tbsp chilli sambal
300ml/1½ pint/1¼ cups coconut milk
350g/12oz/1¼ cups crunchy peanut butter
15ml/1 tbsp dark soy sauce or dark brown sugar
5ml/1 tsp tamarind pulp, soaked in 45ml/3 tbsp warm water
coarsely crushed peanuts
salt

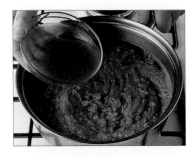

2 Simmer gently until the sauce thickens, then stir in the soy sauce or sugar. Strain in the tamarind juice, add salt to taste and stir well. Spoon into a bowl and sprinkle with a few coarsely crushed peanuts.

Watchpoint

Women who have a history of allergies, or whose partner or family has a history of allergies, are advised to avoid eating peanuts during pregnancy and while breastfeeding.

3 To make the salad, core the cucumber and peel the pears. Cut them into matchsticks. Finely shred the apples and sprinkle them with the lemon juice. Spread a bed of salad leaves on a flat platter, then pile the vegetables and fruit on top. Add the hard-boiled eggs and the chopped noodles. Serve at once, with the sauce.

Nutrition notes

Per portion:

Energy	493Kcals/2061kJ
Protein	18.0g
Fat	34.6g
saturated fat	7.9g
Carbohydrate	29.1g
Fibre	6.7g
Calcium	71.8mg
Folate	55.0µg
Vitamin B$_{12}$	0.3µg
Selenium	4.5µg
Iron	2.4mg
Zinc	2.4mg

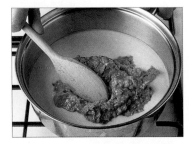

1 Make the peanut sauce. Put the ground chillies or chilli sambal in a pan. Pour in the coconut milk, then stir in the peanut butter. Heat gently, stirring constantly with a wooden spoon, until all the peanut butter has melted and the sauce is smooth.

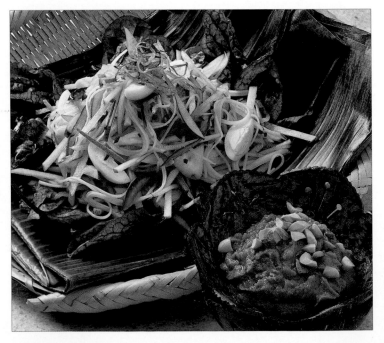

Vegetable salad

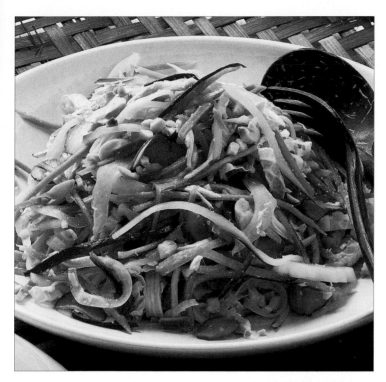

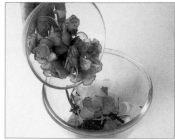

2 Mix together the chilli strips and onion rings in a small bowl. Add the sliced gherkins and lightly ground peanuts and stir to combine.

3 Tip the salted cucumber into a colander, rinse well and drain thoroughly. Using a wooden spatula, press out as much liquid from the cucumber as possible, then pat dry with kitchen paper.

4 Put the cucumber into a salad bowl and add the Chinese leaves and carrot matchsticks. Toss to mix, then add the chilli mixture and slices of cooked chicken.

5 Make a dressing by whisking the gherkin liquid with the garlic, sugar and vinegar in a small bowl or jug (pitcher). Pour over the salad, toss lightly and serve immediately.

High in iron and folates, this salad is perfect to eat throughout pregnancy. It also contains some tangy gherkins, a commonly craved food for pregnant women.

Serves 4

225g/8oz Chinese leaves (cabbage)
2 carrots, cut in matchsticks
½ cucumber, cut in matchsticks
2 fresh red chillies, seeded and cut into thin strips
1 small onion, sliced into fine rings
4 pickled gherkins, sliced, plus 45ml/ 3 tbsp of the liquid
50g/2oz/½ cup peanuts, lightly ground
225g/8oz cooked chicken, finely sliced
1 garlic clove, crushed
5ml/1 tsp granulated sugar
30ml/2 tbsp cider or white vinegar
salt

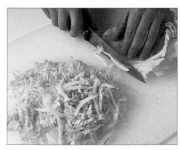

1 Finely slice the Chinese leaves and set aside with the carrot matchsticks. Spread out the cucumber matchsticks on a board and sprinkle with salt. Set aside for 15 minutes.

Watchpoint

If you or your partner suffer from allergies, you should avoid peanuts during pregnancy.

Nutrition notes	
Per portion:	
Energy	183Kcals/765kJ
Protein	18.9g
Fat	8.4g
saturated fat	1.7g
Carbohydrate	8.2g
Fibre	2.9g
Calcium	62.3mg
Folate	73.6µg
Vitamin B$_{12}$	0µg
Selenium	8.4µg
Iron	1.1mg
Zinc	1.1mg

Egg and fennel tabbouleh

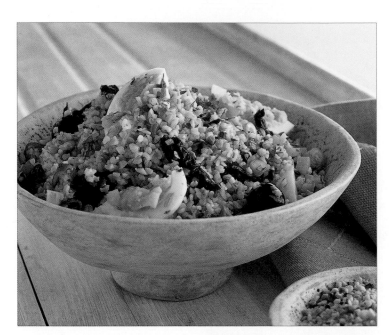

The diverse mix of nutrients provided in this tasty Middle Eastern salad make it a perfect dish to eat from pre-conception right through to breastfeeding.

Serves 4

250g/9oz/1½ cups bulgur wheat
4 small eggs
1 fennel bulb
1 bunch of spring onions (scallions), chopped
25g/1oz/¼ cup drained sun-dried tomatoes in oil, sliced
45ml/3 tbsp chopped fresh flat leaf parsley
30ml/2 tbsp chopped fresh mint
75g/3oz/½ cup black olives
60ml/4 tbsp extra virgin olive oil
30ml/2 tbsp garlic oil
30ml/2 tbsp lemon juice
50g/2oz/½ cup chopped hazelnuts, toasted
salt and ground black pepper
4 pitta breads, warmed, to serve

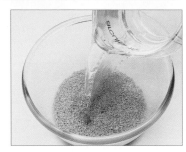

1 Place the bulgur wheat in a large bowl and pour over enough boiling water to cover generously. Leave to soak for about 15 minutes.

Health benefits

Hazelnuts and olives provide a good source of fertility-boosting vitamin E. Garlic contains selenium, another nutrient vital for fertility, while eggs are a staple source of calcium and iron, both of which are important nutrients both during pregnancy and when breastfeeding.

2 Drain the bulgur wheat in a metal sieve (strainer), and place the sieve over a pan of boiling water. Cover the pan and sieve with a lid and steam for about 10 minutes.

3 Remove the lid from the pan and fluff up the grains with a fork. Spread the steamed bulgur wheat out on a metal tray and set aside to cool.

4 Cook the eggs in boiling water for 7–8 minutes. Cool under cold running water, then shell and quarter, or, using an egg slicer, slice not quite all the way through.

5 Halve and finely slice the fennel bulb. Place the pieces in a pan of boiling salted water and cook for about 6 minutes, or until just tender. Drain and cool under running water.

6 Place the eggs, fennel, spring onions, sun-dried tomatoes, parsley, mint and olives in a large salad bowl with the bulgur wheat and toss lightly to mix.

7 Pour over the olive oil, garlic oil and the lemon juice and toss gently until the salad is evenly moist. Sprinkle over the toasted hazelnuts. Season the salad well with salt and ground black pepper and serve with pitta bread.

Nutrition notes	
Per portion:	
Energy	582Kcals/2433kJ
Protein	15.1g
Fat	36.3g
saturated fat	5.1g
Carbohydrate	49.9g
Fibre	2.5g
Calcium	102.7mg
Folate	53.7µg
Vitamin B$_{12}$	0.6µg
Selenium	5.5µg
Iron	5.7mg
Zinc	1.2mg

Warm swordfish and rocket salad

Swordfish is high in the brain-boosting omega-3 fatty acids that are needed by the developing baby in the final trimester. Pecorino cheese is a good source of calcium needed by pregnant women and breastfeeding mothers.

Serves 4

4 swordfish steaks, about 175g/6oz each
75ml/5 tbsp extra virgin olive oil,
     plus extra for serving
juice of 1 lemon
30ml/2 tbsp finely chopped fresh parsley
115g/4oz rocket (arugula) leaves, stalks
     snipped off
115g/4oz Pecorino cheese
salt and ground black pepper

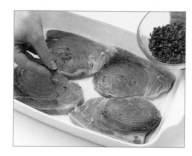

1 Lay the swordfish steaks in a shallow dish large enough to hold them all in a single layer. Mix 60ml/4 tbsp of the olive oil with the lemon juice. Whisk well, then pour the mixture over the fish. Season, sprinkle on the parsley and turn the fish to coat. Cover with plastic wrap and leave at room temperature for 10 minutes.

2 Heat a ridged grilling pan or the grill (broiler) until very hot. Take the fish out of the marinade and pat it dry. Grill or broil for 2–3 minutes on each side until the swordfish is just cooked through, but still juicy.

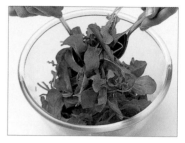

3 Meanwhile, put the rocket leaves in a bowl and season with a little salt and plenty of pepper. Add the remaining 15ml/1 tbsp olive oil and toss. Shave the Pecorino over the top.

4 Place the swordfish steaks on four individual plates and arrange a little pile of salad on each steak. Serve extra olive oil separately so it may be drizzled over the swordfish.

Variation

Oily fish, such as tuna or salmon, would be equally nutritious in this recipe.

Nutrition notes

Per portion:

Energy	451Kcals/1885kJ
Protein	43.6g
Fat	30.5g
saturated fat	9.5g
Carbohydrate	0.5g
Fibre	0.6g
Calcium	400mg
Folate	46.8µg
Vitamin B_{12}	7.5µg
Selenium	82.5µg
Iron	1.8mg
Zinc	1.7mg

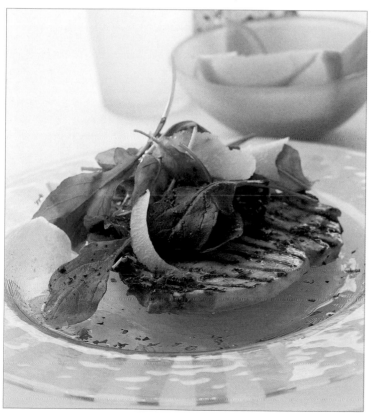

Salad nicoise

This tuna and egg salad is a great all-round dish for pre-conception through to breastfeeding, as it provides valuable supplies of folates, omega-3 fatty acids, iron and calcium.

Serves 4

115g/4oz French (green) beans, trimmed and cut in half
115g/4oz mixed salad leaves
½ small cucumber, thinly sliced
4 ripe tomatoes, quartered
1 tuna steak, about 175g/6oz in weight
olive oil, for brushing
4 eggs, hard-boiled (hard-cooked)
50g/2oz can anchovies, drained and halved lengthways
½ bunch small radishes, trimmed
50g/2oz/½cup small black olives
salt and ground black pepper

For the dressing
90ml/6 tbsp extra virgin olive oil
2 garlic cloves, crushed
15ml/1 tbsp white wine vinegar

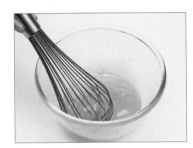

1 To make the dressing, whisk together the oil, garlic and vinegar and season to taste with salt and black pepper. Set aside until ready to use.

2 Cook the French beans in a pan of boiling water for 2 minutes until just tender, then drain.

3 Mix together the salad leaves, sliced cucumber, tomatoes and French beans in a large, shallow bowl.

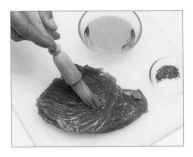

4 Preheat the grill (broiler). Brush the tuna steak with olive oil and sprinkle with salt and ground black pepper.

5 Grill (broil) for 3–4 minutes on each side until cooked through. Allow to cool, then gently flake with a fork. Shell the hard-boiled eggs and cut them into quarters, or slice thickly.

6 Scatter the flaked tuna, anchovies, eggs, radishes and olives over the salad. Pour over the dressing and toss together lightly. Serve at once.

Nutrition notes	
Per portion:	
Energy	352Kcals/1471kJ
Protein	21.3g
Fat	28.2g
saturated fat	4.7g
Carbohydrate	3.7g
Fibre	2.0g
Calcium	107mg
Folate	81.7µg
Vitamin B$_{12}$	3.7µg
Selenium	30.9µg
Iron	3.1mg
Zinc	1.5mg

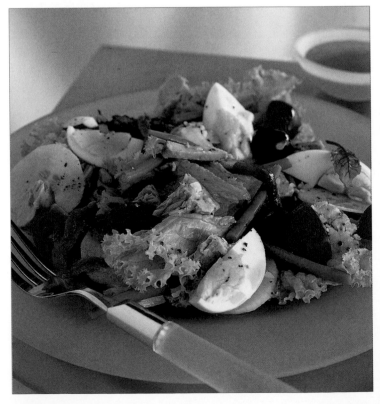

Rice pilaff with fruit and nuts

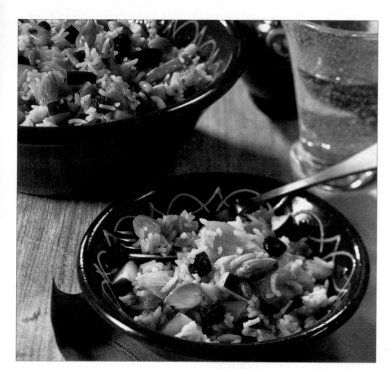

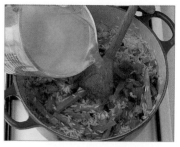

3 Add the stock, orange juice and rind, stirring. Reserve a few toasted almonds and stir in the rest with the pine nuts.

4 Cover the pan with double foil and a tight-fitting lid. Bake in the oven for 30–35 minutes, until the rice is tender and all the liquid has been absorbed.

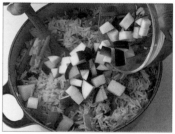

5 Cool slightly, then season well. Stir in the chopped apple and serve garnished with the reserved almonds.

This colourful rice dish is rich in vitamin E and iron. It's a fuss-free meal, since after the initial quick cook it is baked in the oven.

Serves 4

60ml/4 tbsp sunflower oil
75g/3oz/¾ cup blanched almonds
225g/8oz carrots, cut into fine julienne strips
2 onions, chopped
115g/4oz/½ cup ready-to-eat dried apricots, chopped
50g/2oz/⅓ cup raisins
350g/12oz/1¾cups basmati rice, soaked and drained
600ml/1 pint/2½ cups vegetable stock
150ml/¼ pint/⅔ cup orange juice
grated rind of 1 orange
25g/1oz/⅓ cup pine nuts
1 red eating apple, chopped
salt and ground black pepper

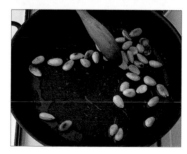

1 Preheat the oven to 160°C/325°F/ Gas 3. Heat a little of the oil in a pan and fry the almonds until golden.

2 Heat the remaining oil in a heavy, flameproof casserole and fry the carrots and onions over a moderately high heat for 6–8 minutes until slightly glazed. Add the apricots, raisins and rice and cook over a medium heat for a few minutes, stirring all the time, until the grains of rice are coated in the oil.

Nutrition notes	
Per portion:	
Energy	676Kcals/2626kJ
Protein	13.2g
Fat	26.7g
saturated fat	2.5g
Carbohydrate	96.3g
Fibre	4.7g
Calcium	110mg
Folate	45.4µg
Vitamin B$_{12}$	0.0µg
Selenium	3.5µg
Iron	3.2mg
Zinc	1.4mg

Frittata with leeks, pepper and spinach

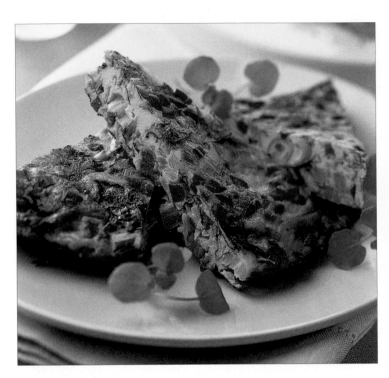

This is a perfect pre-pregnancy dish, rich in sperm-boosting vitamin E and full of valuable folates, which are so essential before conception and during the first 12 weeks of pregnancy.

Serves 3-4

30ml/2 tbsp olive oil
1 large red (bell) pepper, seeded and diced
2.5–5ml/½ –1 tsp toasted cumin seeds, ground
3 leeks (about 450g/1lb), thinly sliced
150g/5oz small spinach leaves
45ml/3 tbsp pine nuts, toasted
5 large eggs
15ml/1 tbsp chopped fresh basil
15ml/1 tbsp chopped fresh flat leaf parsley
salt and ground black pepper
watercress, rocket (arugula) or other salad leaves, to garnish

1 Heat a frying pan and add the oil. Add the red pepper and cook over a medium heat, stirring, for 6–8 minutes, until soft and beginning to brown. Add 2.5ml/½ tsp of the cumin, stir well and cook for another 1–2 minutes.

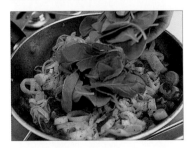

2 Stir in the leeks, then partially cover the pan and cook gently for about 5 minutes, until the leeks have softened and collapsed. Season with salt and ground black pepper. Place the spinach on top and cover the pan.

3 Allow the spinach to wilt in the steam for 3–4 minutes, then stir to mix it into the vegetables. Stir in the pine nuts.

4 Beat the eggs in a bowl with salt, pepper and the remaining cumin. Stir in the chopped basil and parsley.

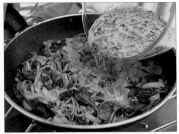

5 Pour the egg mixture into the pan. Cook over a gentle heat until the bottom of the omelette sets and turns golden brown. Pull the edges of the omelette away from the sides of the pan as it cooks, and tilt the pan so that the uncooked egg runs underneath.

6 Preheat the grill (broiler). Put the frittata under the hot grill to set the egg on top and ensure that it is cooked throughout, but do not let it become too brown. Cut the frittata into wedges and serve warm, garnished with watercress or other green salad leaves.

Nutrition notes	
Per portion:	
Energy	265Kcals/1045kJ
Protein	12.6g
Fat	20.9g
saturated fat	3.4g
Carbohydrate	6.8g
Fibre	4.1g
Calcium	130mg
Folate	152µg
Vitamin B$_{12}$	0.7µg
Selenium	8.4µg
Iron	3.9mg
Zinc	2.1mg

Vegetable pancakes with tomato salsa

These little spinach and egg pancakes contain folates, essential fatty acids and calcium, making them ideal from pre-conception through to breastfeeding.

Serves 4

225g/8oz spinach
1 small leek
a few sprigs of fresh coriander (cilantro) or parsley
3 large eggs
50g/2oz/½ cup plain (all-purpose) flour, sifted
salt, ground black pepper and grated nutmeg, to taste
olive oil, for frying
25g/1oz/⅓ cup freshly grated Parmesan cheese, for sprinkling

For the tomato salsa
2 tomatoes, peeled and chopped
¼ fresh red chilli, finely chopped
2 pieces sun-dried tomato in oil, drained and chopped
1 small red onion, chopped
1 garlic clove, crushed
60ml/4 tbsp extra virgin olive oil
30ml/2 tbsp sherry
2.5ml/½ tsp soft light brown sugar

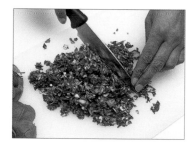

1 Finely chop the spinach with the leek and coriander or parsley. Use a food processor if you like, but do not over-process; the mixture must not form a paste. Transfer to a large bowl.

2 Beat the eggs in to the spinach and add seasoning to taste. Gradually blend in the flour and 30–45ml/2–3 tbsp water and set aside for 20 minutes.

3 Make the salsa. Mix together all the ingredients in a bowl, then cover and set aside for 2–3 hours.

Nutrition notes

Per pancake:

Energy	69Kcals/289kJ
Protein	4g
Fat	4.1g
saturated fat	1.1g
Carbohydrate	4.6g
Fibre	0.7g
Calcium	75.1mg
Folate	43.7µg
Vitamin B_{12}	0.5µg
Selenium	2.5µg
Iron	0.9mg
Zinc	0.5mg

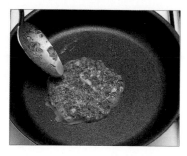

4 Heat a lightly oiled, non-stick frying pan, then drop in small spoonfuls of the batter and fry until golden underneath. Turn and cook briefly on the other side. Drain on kitchen paper and keep warm. Sprinkle with a little grated Parmesan and serve hot with the spicy tomato salsa.

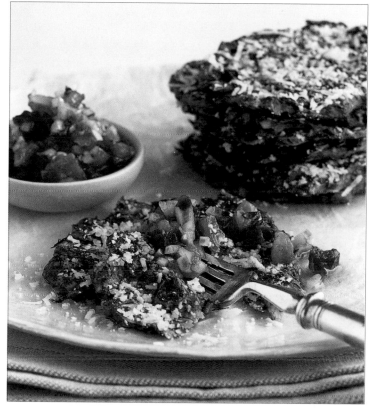

Fish and vegetable stir-fry

This light dish is ideal for early pregnancy. The ginger is great for nausea, and mangetouts, sweetcorn and asparagus are packed with folates. Nutritious light meals like this are also great later in pregnancy if larger meals cause indigestion.

Serves 4

675g/1½lb cod or hoki fillet, skinned
pinch of five-spice powder
2 carrots
115g/4oz/1 cup small mangetouts (snow peas)
115g/4oz asparagus spears
4 spring onions (scallions)
8–12 small baby corn cobs
45ml/3 tbsp groundnut or stir-fry oil
2.5cm/1in piece fresh root ginger, peeled and cut into thin slivers
2 garlic cloves, finely chopped
300g/11oz beansprouts
15–30ml/1–2 tbsp light soy sauce
salt and ground black pepper

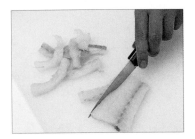

1 Cut the fish fillets into finger-size strips and season lightly with salt, pepper and five-spice powder. Cut the carrots diagonally into slices that are as thin as the mangetouts.

2 Top and tail the mangetouts. Trim the asparagus spears and cut in half crossways. Trim the spring onions and cut them diagonally into 2cm/¾in pieces, keeping the white and green parts separate. Mix together the carrots, mangetouts, asparagus and corn in a bowl and set them aside.

3 Heat the oil in a wok. Stir-fry the ginger and garlic for 1 minute, then add the white parts of the spring onions and cook for 1 minute more.

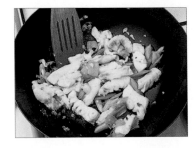

4 Add the fish strips and stir-fry for 2–3 minutes, until opaque. Add the beansprouts, toss well, then add the carrots, mangetouts, asparagus and corn. Stir-fry for 3–4 minutes.

5 Stir in light soy sauce to taste and toss to combine. Add the green parts of the spring onions to the pan and stir. Serve with rice or noodles.

Nutrition notes	
Per portion:	
Energy	185Kcals/773kJ
Protein	22.4g
Fat	8.2g
saturated fat	1g
Carbohydrate	5.7g
Fibre	2.6g
Calcium	62.8mg
Folate	313.9µg
Vitamin B$_{12}$	0µg
Selenium	47.6µg
Iron	2.3mg
Zinc	0.9mg

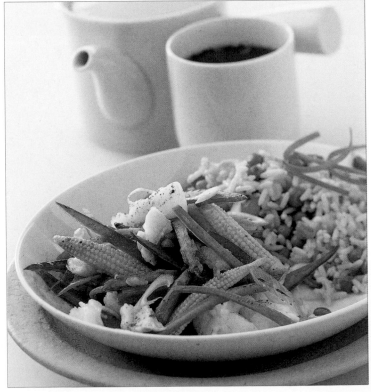

Tagliatelle with spinach and broccoli

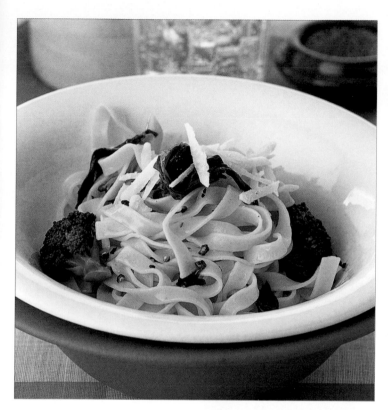

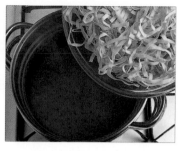

2 Top up the water in the steamer pan and add salt. Bring to the boil, then cook the pasta until just tender. Meanwhile, cut the broccoli into florets and coarsley chop the spinach.

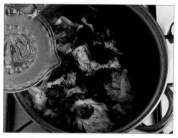

3 Drain the pasta. Heat the oil in the pasta pan, then add the pasta and chopped vegetables and toss well. Add lemon juice and black pepper to taste, then serve immediately with the grated Parmesan cheese.

Broccoli and spinach are packed with vital folates, which are essential in early pregnancy. If you're suffering from morning sickness, you may wish to reduce the amount of oil that is mixed in with the pasta.

Serves 4

2 heads of broccoli
450g/1lb fresh spinach, stalks and any coarse
  leaves removed
nutmeg
450g/1lb fresh or dried egg tagliatelle
about 45ml/3 tbsp extra virgin olive oil
juice of ½ lemon, or to taste
salt and ground black pepper
freshly grated Parmesan cheese, to serve

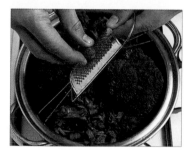

1 Remove the thick stalk from the broccoli and steam over boiling water for 10 minutes. Add the spinach to the broccoli, cover and steam for 4–5 minutes or until both are tender. Towards the end of the cooking time, grate fresh nutmeg over the vegetables and add salt and pepper to taste. Transfer the vegetables to a colander.

Nutrition notes	
Per portion:	
Energy	583Kcals/2437kJ
Protein	22.3g
Fat	19.5g
saturated fat	4.1g
Carbohydrate	84.7g
Fibre	8.9g
Calcium	292mg
Folate	313.9µg
Vitamin B$_{12}$	0µg
Selenium	1.1µg
Iron	6.2mg
Zinc	3mg

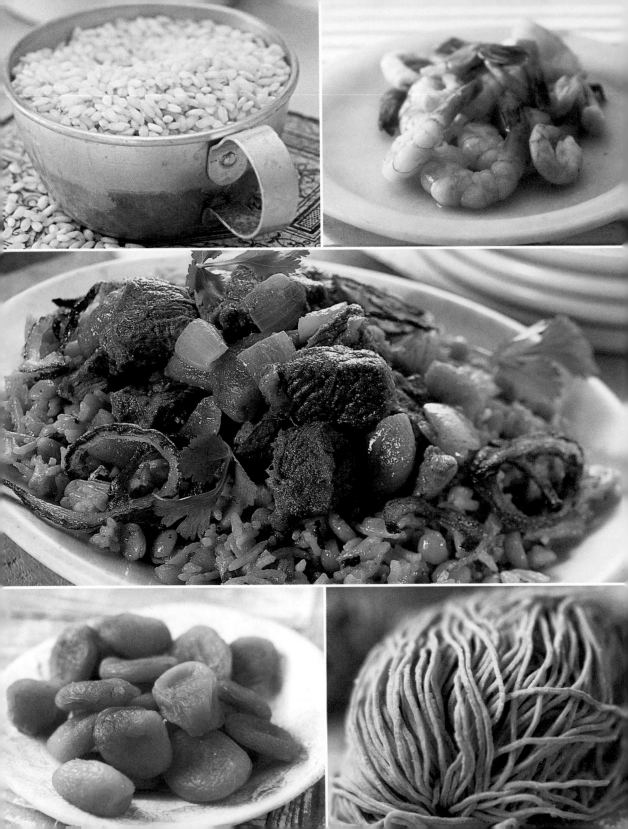

main meals

This chapter includes a range of dishes that are
perfect for eating from pre-conception through to pregnancy.
The foods they contain can help with fertility, promote healthy
foetal development and provide new mothers with the nutrients
they need for breastfeeding. Moroccan Paella can boost fertility,
Bacon-wrapped Trout with Oatmeal Stuffing provides
brain-growing omega-3 fatty acids, and Beef and Vegetable
Stir-fry is rich in iron for later in pregnancy and after the birth.

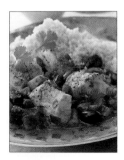
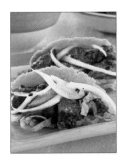
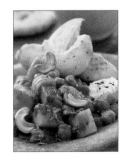

Seared tuna with red onion salsa

Tuna is a good source of omega-3 fatty acids, which are needed for brain growth in the second and third trimesters. The salsa contains fertility-boosting vitamin E, as well as folates for pre-conception and the first trimester.

Serves 4

4 tuna steaks, each weighing about
    175–200g/6–7oz
5ml/1 tsp cumin seeds, toasted
    and crushed
pinch of dried red chilli flakes
grated rind and juice of 1 lime
30–60ml/2–4 tbsp extra virgin olive oil
salt and ground black pepper
lime wedges and fresh coriander (cilantro)
    sprigs, to garnish

For the salsa

1 small red onion, finely chopped
200g/7oz red or yellow cherry tomatoes,
    roughly chopped
1 avocado, peeled, stoned and chopped
2 kiwi fruit, peeled and chopped
1 fresh red chilli, seeded and finely
    chopped
15g/½oz fresh coriander (cilantro), chopped
6 fresh mint sprigs, leaves only, chopped
5ml/1 tsp Thai fish sauce (nam pla)
5ml/1 tsp muscovado (molasses) sugar

Nutrition notes	
Per portion:	
Energy	433Kcals/1810kJ
Protein	49g
Fat	23.5g
saturated fat	5.3g
Carbohydrate	6.7g
Fibre	2.7g
Calcium	53.6mg
Folate	44.5µg
Vitamin B$_{12}$	8µg
Selenium	114µg
Iron	3.1mg
Zinc	1.7mg

1 Sprinkle the tuna steaks with half the cumin, the dried chilli, salt, pepper and half the lime rind. Rub in 30ml/2 tbsp of the oil and set aside for about 30 minutes.

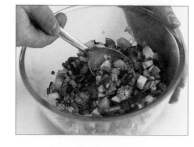

2 Make the salsa by mixing all the ingredients in a bowl. Add the remaining cumin, the rest of the lime rind and half the lime juice. Set aside for 15–20 minutes, then add more Thai fish sauce, lime juice and olive oil if required.

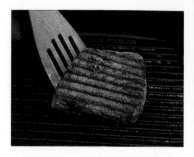

3 Heat a ridged, cast-iron griddle or grill pan. Cook the prepared tuna steaks, allowing 2 minutes on each side for rare tuna or a little longer for a medium result.

4 Serve the tuna steaks garnished with lime wedges and coriander sprigs. Serve the salsa separately or spoon a little on to each plate, with the tuna.

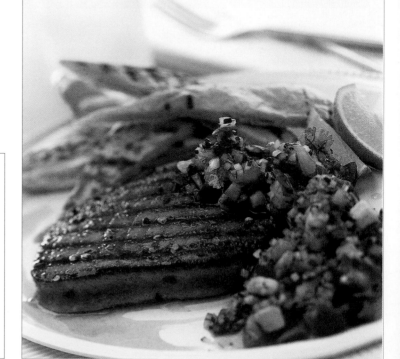

Bacon-wrapped trout with oatmeal stuffing

Trout is an excellent source of brain-boosting omega-3 fatty acids, and the oatmeal stuffing provides valuable extra fibre, which is important during pregnancy. This dish also contains a good supply of iron, which is essential both later in pregnancy and when breastfeeding.

Serves 4

10 dry-cured streaky (fatty) bacon rashers
45ml/3 tbsp olive oil
1 onion, finely chopped
115g/4oz/1 cup oatmeal
30ml/2 tbsp chopped fresh parsley
30ml/2 tbsp snipped fresh chives
4 trout, about 350g/12oz each, gutted and boned
juice of ½ lemon
salt and ground black pepper
watercress, cherry tomatoes and lemon wedges,
    to serve

For the herb mayonnaise
6 watercress sprigs
15ml/1 tbsp snipped fresh chives
30ml/2 tbsp roughly chopped parsley
90ml/6 tbsp lemon mayonnaise
30ml/2 tbsp fromage frais, ricotta cheese or
    crème fraîche
2.5–5ml/½–1 tsp tarragon mustard

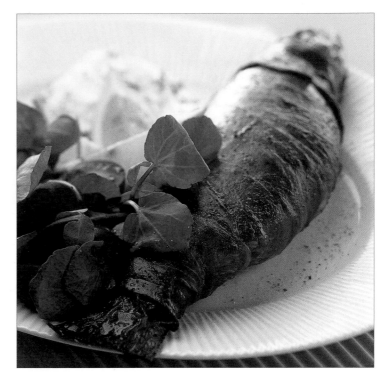

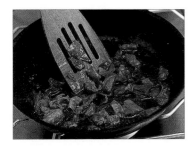

1 Preheat the oven to 190ºC/375ºF/Gas 5. Chop two of the bacon rashers. Heat 30ml/2 tbsp of the oil in a large frying pan and cook the bacon briefly. Add the finely chopped onion and fry gently for 5–8 minutes, until softened.

2 Add the oatmeal and cook until it darkens and absorbs the oil; do not let it over-brown. Stir in the herbs and seasoning. Cool.

3 Wash and dry the trout, then stuff with the oatmeal mixture. Wrap each fish in two bacon rashers and place in an ovenproof dish. Sprinkle with the remaining oil and the lemon juice. Bake for 20–25 minutes.

4 Meanwhile, make the mayonnaise. Place the watercress and herbs in a sieve and pour boiling water over them. Drain, rinse under cold water, and drain on kitchen paper.

5 Pound the herbs in a mortar with a pestle to form a paste, then stir into the lemon mayonnaise with the fromage frais, ricotta or crème fraîche. Stir in tarragon mustard to taste.

6 When the fish are cooked, and the bacon is slightly crisp, transfer them to warmed serving plates. Serve immediately with watercress, tomatoes and lemon wedges, accompanied by the herb mayonnaise.

Nutrition notes	
Per portion:	
Energy	868Kcals/3628kJ
Protein	68.8g
Fat	55.5g
saturated fat	11.5g
Carbohydrate	24.7g
Fibre	2.5g
Calcium	89.6mg
Folate	51.2µg
Vitamin B$_{12}$	14.9µg
Selenium	57.9µg
Iron	2.7mg
Zinc	3.3mg

Filipino spinach and fish stew

This is a great pre-pregnancy dish, which is low in fat and high in valuable protein.

Serves 4

15ml/1 tbsp tamarind pulp
150ml/¼ pint/⅔ cup warm water
2 tomatoes
115g/4oz spinach
115g/4oz cooked large prawns (jumbo shrimp),
  thawed if frozen
1.2 litres/2 pints/5 cups fish stock
½ mooli (daikon), peeled and finely diced
115g/4oz French (green) beans,
  cut into 1cm/½in lengths
225g/8oz piece of cod or haddock fillet, skinned
  and cut into strips
fish sauce, to taste
squeeze of lemon juice, to taste
salt and ground black pepper
boiled rice or noodles, to serve

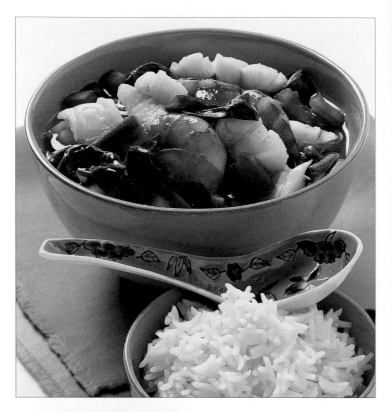

1 Put the tamarind pulp in a bowl and pour over the warm water. Set aside while you peel and chop the tomatoes, discarding the seeds. Strip the spinach leaves from the stems and tear them into small pieces. Set aside.

2 Remove the heads and shells from the prawns, leaving the tail shells intact, if you like.

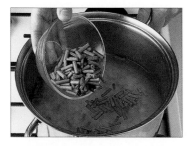

3 Bring the fish stock to the boil in a large pan, add the diced mooli and cook for 5 minutes, then add the beans and continue to cook for another 3–5 minutes.

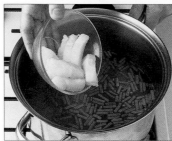

4 Add the fish strips, diced tomato and spinach. Strain in the tamarind juice and cook for 2 minutes.

5 Stir the cooked prawns into the stew and cook for 1–2 minutes, until they are just heated through. Do not let them overcook or they will become tough.

6 Season the stew and add fish sauce and lemon juice to taste. Ladle into individual serving bowls and serve immediately, with rice or noodles.

Nutrition notes	
Per portion:	
Energy	62Kcals/259kJ
Protein	11.4g
Fat	0.7g
saturated fat	0.1g
Carbohydrate	2.3g
Fibre	1.1g
Calcium	65.1mg
Folate	60µg
Vitamin B$_{12}$	1.7µg
Selenium	13.7µg
Iron	1.2mg
Zinc	0.7mg

Teriyaki soba noodles with beancurd

This healthy, nutritious dish is very quick to cook and combines noodles, fresh vegetables and tofu with a piquant sauce to provide a range of nutrients for every stage of your pregnancy.

Serves 4

350g/12oz soba noodles
30ml/2 tbsp toasted sesame oil
200g/7oz asparagus tips
30ml/2 tbsp groundnut (peanut) or vegetable oil
225g/8oz block of beancurd (tofu)
2 spring onions (scallions), cut into thin strips
1 carrot, cut into matchsticks
2.5ml/½ tsp chilli flakes
15ml/1 tbsp sesame seeds
salt and freshly ground black pepper

For the teriyaki sauce
60ml/4 tbsp dark soy sauce
60ml/4 tbsp Japanese saké, dry sherry or dry vermouth
60ml/4 tbsp mirin
5ml/1 tsp caster (superfine) sugar

1 Cook the noodles in boiling salted water according to the instructions on the packet, then drain and rinse under cold running water. Set aside.

2 Heat the sesame oil in a griddle pan or in a baking sheet placed under the grill (broiler) until very hot. Turn down the heat to medium, then cook the asparagus for 8–10 minutes, turning frequently, until tender and browned. Set aside.

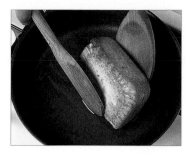

3 Meanwhile, heat the groundnut or vegetable oil in a wok or large frying pan until very hot. Add the beancurd and fry for 8–10 minutes until golden, turning it occasionally to crisp all sides. Carefully lift it out and drain on kitchen paper. Cut the beancurd into 1cm/½in slices.

4 To prepare the teriyaki sauce, mix the ingredients together, then heat the mixture in the wok or frying pan.

5 Toss in the noodles and stir to coat. Heat through for 1–2 minutes, then spoon into individual bowls, with the tofu and asparagus. Scatter the spring onions and carrot on top and sprinkle with the chilli flakes and sesame seeds. Serve.

Nutrition notes	
Per portion:	
Energy	476Kcals/1990kJ
Protein	10.5g
Fat	13.8g
saturated fat	1.7g
Carbohydrate	74.4g
Fibre	1.5g
Calcium	326mg
Folate	102.9µg
Vitamin B$_{12}$	0µg
Selenium	0.7µg
Iron	2.6mg
Zinc	0.8mg

Health benefits

Beancurd is the perfect food for pregnancy. It contains vitamin E to boost fertility before conception, essential fatty acids to help your baby's brain grow, and calcium and iron, which are needed during pregnancy and while breastfeeding.

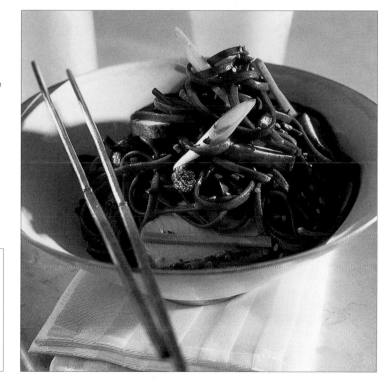

Fish tagine

This dish contains valuable nutrients needed during pregnancy, for baby's growing brain.

Serves 8

1.3kg/3lb firm fish fillets, skinned and cut into 5cm/2in chunks
60ml/4 tbsp extra virgin olive oil
4 onions, chopped
1 large aubergine (eggplant), cut into 1cm/½in cubes
2 courgettes (zucchini), cut into 1cm/½in cubes
400g/14oz can chopped tomatoes
400ml/14fl oz/1⅔ cups passata (puréed tomatoes)
200ml/7fl oz/scant 1 cup fish stock
1 preserved lemon, chopped
90g/3½oz/scant 1 cup pitted black or green olives
60ml/4 tbsp chopped fresh coriander (cilantro), plus extra to garnish
salt and ground black pepper

For the harissa
3 large fresh red chillies, seeded and chopped
3 garlic cloves, peeled
15ml/1 tbsp ground coriander
30ml/2 tbsp ground cumin
5ml/1 tsp ground cinnamon
grated rind of 1 lemon
30ml/2 tbsp sunflower oil

1 To make the harissa, place all the ingredients in a food processor or blender and process to a smooth paste.

2 Put the chunks of fish in a wide bowl and add 30ml/2 tbsp of the harissa. Toss to coat, cover and chill for at least 1 hour, or overnight.

3 Heat half the oil in a shallow, heavy pan. Cook the onions gently for 10 minutes, until golden brown. Stir in the remaining harissa; cook for 5 minutes, stirring the mixture occasionally.

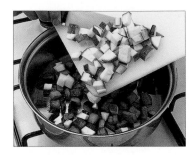

4 Heat the remaining olive oil in a separate pan. Add the aubergine cubes and fry, stirring occasionally, for about 10 minutes, until they are golden brown. Add the cubed courgettes and fry for a further 2 minutes.

5 Tip the mixture into the onions and combine, then stir in the chopped tomatoes, the passata and fish stock. Bring to the boil, then simmer for about 20 minutes.

6 Stir in the fish chunks, preserved lemon and olives. Cover and simmer for 15–20 minutes until the fish is just cooked through. Season to taste. Stir in the chopped coriander. Serve with couscous, if you like, and garnish with a few coriander sprigs.

Nutrition notes	
Per portion:	
Energy	254Kcals/1062kJ
Protein	34.2g
Fat	9.6g
saturated fat	1.4g
Carbohydrate	8.1g
Fibre	2.2g
Calcium	54.8mg
Folate	55.7µg
Vitamin B_{12}	1.8µg
Selenium	49.6µg
Iron	1.1mg
Zinc	1mg

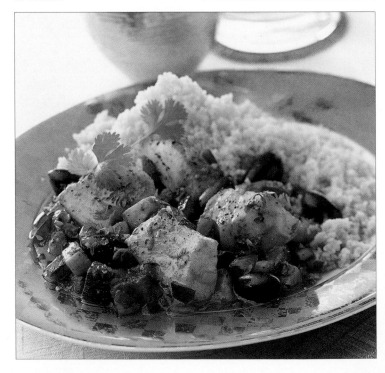

Moroccan paella

Shellfish are a good source of zinc and selenium, but make sure the mussels are thoroughly cooked.

Serves 6

2 large skinless, boneless chicken breasts
about 150g/5oz prepared squid, cut into rings
275/10oz cod or haddock fillets, skinned and cut into bite-size chunks
8–10 raw king prawns (jumbo shrimp), peeled and deveined
8 scallops, trimmed and halved
350g/12oz mussels, scrubbed and bearded
250g/9oz/1⅓ cups long grain rice
30ml/2 tbsp sunflower oil
1 bunch spring onions (scallions), cut into strips
2 small courgettes (zucchini), cut into strips
1 red (bell) pepper, cored, seeded and cut into strips
400ml/14fl oz/1⅔cups chicken stock
250ml/8fl oz/1 cup passata (puréed tomatoes)
salt and freshly ground black pepper
fresh coriander (cilantro) sprigs and lemon wedges, to garnish (optional)

For the marinade
2 fresh red chillies, seeded and roughly chopped
generous handful of fresh coriander (cilantro)
10–15ml/2–3 tsp ground cumin
15ml/1 tbsp paprika
2 garlic cloves
45ml/3 tbsp olive oil
60ml/4 tbsp sunflower oil
juice of 1 lemon

1 Process all the ingredients for the marinade in a food processor with 5ml/1 tsp salt. Cut the chicken into bitesize pieces. Place in a bowl.

2 Place the fish and shellfish (not the mussels) in a separate bowl. Divide the marinade between the chicken and fish, then stir. Cover and leave for 2 hours.

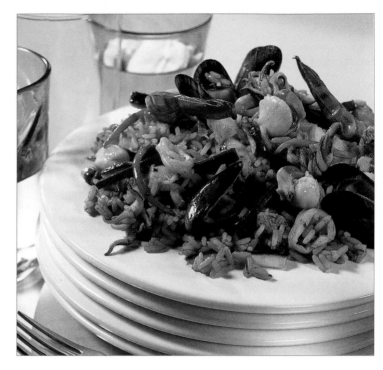

3 Place the rice in a bowl, pour over enough boiling water to cover and set aside for 30 minutes. Drain the chicken and fish, reserving the marinade. Heat the oil in a wok and fry the chicken for a few minutes until lightly browned.

4 Add the spring onions to the pan, fry for 1 minute and then add the courgettes and red pepper and fry for 3–4 minutes more. Transfer the chicken and the vegetables to separate plates.

5 Scrape the marinade into the pan and cook for 1 minute. Drain the rice, add to the pan and cook for a further minute. Add the chicken stock, passata and chicken, season and stir. Bring to the boil, cover, and simmer for 10–15 minutes.

6 Add the cooked vegetables to the pan and place all the fish and mussels on top.

7 Cover again with a lid or foil and cook over a moderate heat for 10–12 minutes until the fish is cooked and the mussels have opened. Discard any mussels that remain closed. Serve immediately, garnished with fresh coriander and lemon wedges, if liked.

Nutrition notes	
Per portion:	
Energy	467Kcals/1952kJ
Protein	46.4g
Fat	13.8g
saturated fat	2.3g
Carbohydrate	42.1g
Fibre	1.5g
Calcium	116mg
Folate	84.7µg
Vitamin B$_{12}$	15.5µg
Selenium	84.6mg
Iron	5.4mg
Zinc	4.1mg

Watchpoint

Mussels are a common source of food poisoning so should be avoided during pregnancy.

Spiced vegetable couscous

This hearty stew is flavoured with a blend of aromatic spices and is great to eat at any time during pregnancy.

Serves 6

30ml/2 tbsp extra virgin olive oil
1 large onion, finely chopped
2 garlic cloves, crushed
15ml/1 tbsp tomato purée (paste)
2.5ml/½ tsp ground turmeric
2.5ml/½ tsp cayenne pepper
5ml/1 tsp ground coriander
5ml/1 tsp ground cumin
225g/8oz/1½ cups cauliflower florets
225g/8oz baby carrots, trimmed
1 red (bell) pepper, seeded and diced
4 beefsteak tomatoes
225g/8oz courgettes (zucchini), thickly
  sliced
400g/14oz can chickpeas, drained
  and rinsed
45ml/3 tbsp chopped fresh coriander (cilantro),
  plus a few extra sprigs to garnish
salt and ground black pepper

For the couscous
30ml/2 tbsp extra virgin olive oil
5ml/1 tsp salt
450g/1lb/2⅔ cups couscous

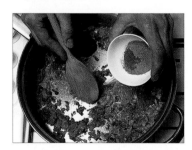

1 Heat the olive oil in a large pan, add the onion and garlic, and cook for 5 minutes, stirring occasionally, or until the onion is softened. Stir in the tomato purée, turmeric, cayenne, ground coriander and cumin. Cook, stirring, for about 2 minutes.

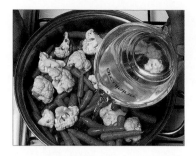

2 Add the cauliflower florets, baby carrots and red pepper to the pan, with enough water to come halfway up the vegetables. Bring to the boil, then lower the heat, cover and simmer for about 10 minutes.

3 Plunge the tomatoes into boiling water for 30 seconds, then refresh in cold water.

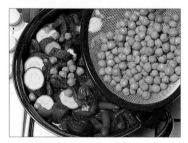

4 Peel away the skins from the tomatoes and chop the flesh roughly. Add the sliced courgettes, chickpeas and tomatoes to the other vegetables and cook for a further 10 minutes. Stir in the chopped fresh coriander and season with plenty of salt and ground black pepper. Keep hot.

Health benefits
Chickpeas are a great food to eat during pregnancy. They contain a rich supply of folates, important for pre-conception and the first 12 weeks of pregnancy, and they are also high in iron, which is essential later in pregnancy and after the birth.

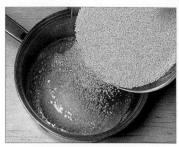

5 To cook the couscous, bring 475ml/16fl oz/2 cups water to the boil in a large pan. Add about half the olive oil and the salt. Remove the pan from the heat, and pour in the couscous, stirring all the time. Set the pan aside and leave the couscous to absorb the water for about 2 minutes.

6 When all of the water has been absorbed, add the remaining olive oil to the couscous. Place the pan over a low heat and heat the couscous through gently, stirring occasionally to separate and fluff the grains.

7 As soon as it has warmed through, tip out the couscous on to a warm serving dish or divide among individual bowls. Spoon the spiced vegetables on top, pouring over any liquid, then garnish with fresh coriander sprigs and serve immediately.

Nutrition notes	
Per portion:	
Energy	368Kcals/1538kJ
Protein	12.7g
Fat	9.3g
saturated fat	1.3g
Carbohydrate	61.9g
Fibre	6.6g
Calcium	88.6mg
Folate	85.5µg
Vitamin B$_{12}$	0µg
Selenium	1.8µg
Iron	6.2mg
Zinc	1.1mg

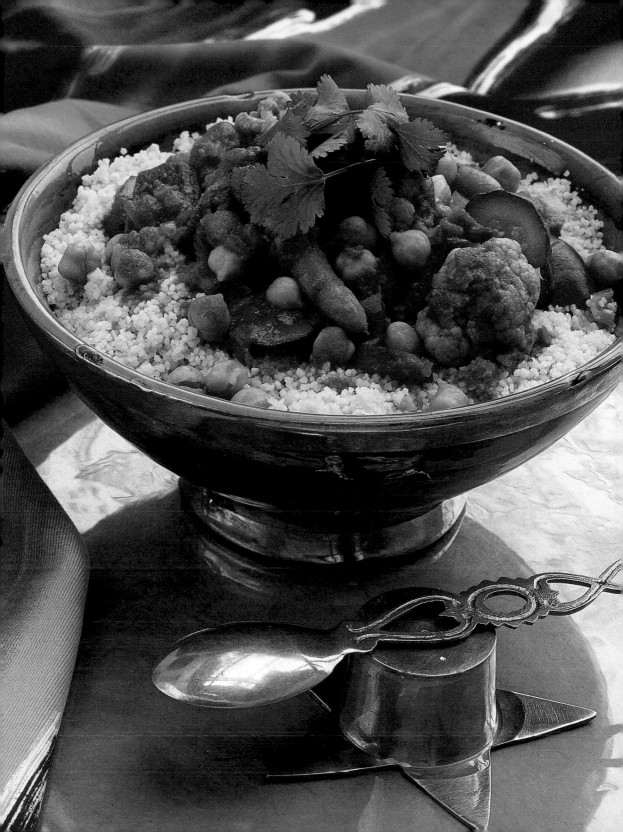

Egg and lentil curry

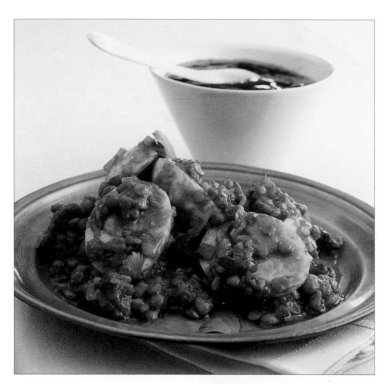

This dish is a useful source of folates, calcium, iron and zinc, so is good any time from pre-conception to breastfeeding.

Serves 4

75g/3oz/scant ½ cup green lentils
750ml/1¼ pints/3 cups vegetable stock
6 eggs
30ml/2 tbsp sunflower oil
3 cloves
1.5ml/¼ tsp black peppercorns
1 onion, finely chopped
2 fresh green chillies, finely chopped
2 garlic cloves, crushed
2.5cm/1in piece fresh root ginger, chopped
30ml/2 tbsp curry paste
400g/14oz can chopped tomatoes
2.5ml/½ tsp granulated sugar
2.5ml/½ tsp garam masala

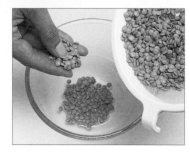

1 Wash the lentils, then put them in a heavy pan with the stock. Cover and bring to the boil. Reduce the heat and simmer for 15 minutes or until the lentils are soft. Drain and set aside.

Watchpoint

When you are pregnant, always make sure that eggs are thoroughly cooked.

---

2 Cook the eggs in boiling water for 7–10 minutes. Remove from the pan and set aside to cool slightly.

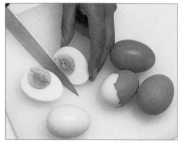

3 When the eggs are cool enough to handle, peel them and then cut in half lengthways.

4 Heat the oil in a large frying pan and fry the cloves and peppercorns, stirring, for 2 minutes. Add the onion, chillies, garlic and ginger and fry for 5–6 minutes, stirring frequently. Stir in the curry paste and fry for a further 2 minutes, stirring constantly.

5 Add the chopped tomatoes and sugar and stir in 175ml/6fl oz/¾ cup water. Simmer for about 5 minutes until the sauce thickens, stirring occasionally. Add the halved eggs, drained lentils and garam masala. Cover and simmer for a further 10 minutes, then serve.

Nutrition notes	
Per portion:	
Energy	262Kcals/1095kJ
Protein	15.7g
Fat	15.7g
saturated fat	3g
Carbohydrate	15.6g
Fibre	2.9g
Calcium	88.7mg
Folate	67.2µg
Vitamin B_{12}	0.8µg
Selenium	28.1µg
Iron	4.9mg
Zinc	1.9mg

Spicy parsnips and chickpeas in ginger

Don't be put off by the long list of ingredients, as this tasty vegetarian stew is surprisingly easy to cook. It contains folates, which means that it is good to eat before conception and during early pregnancy. High in iron, it is excellent to eat later in pregnancy, too.

Serves 4

200g/7oz dried chickpeas, soaked overnight in
    cold water, then drained
7 garlic cloves, finely chopped
1 small onion, chopped
5cm/2in piece fresh root ginger, chopped
2 fresh green chillies, seeded and
    finely chopped
550ml/18fl oz/2½ cups water
60ml/4 tbsp groundnut (peanut) oil
5ml/1 tsp cumin seeds
10ml/2 tsp ground coriander seeds
5ml/1 tsp ground turmeric
2.5–5ml/½–1 tsp chilli powder
50g/2oz cashew nuts, toasted and ground
250g/9oz tomatoes, peeled and chopped
900g/2lb parsnips, cut into chunks
5ml/1 tsp ground roasted cumin seeds
juice of 1 lime, to taste (optional)
salt and ground black pepper
fresh coriander (cilantro) leaves, natural (plain)
    yogurt, and a few cashew nuts, toasted,
    to serve

1 Put the soaked chickpeas in a pan, cover with water and bring to the boil. Boil vigorously for 10 minutes, then reduce the heat so that the water boils steadily and cook for 1–1½ hours, or until the chickpeas are tender. Drain.

2 Set 10ml/2 tsp of the garlic aside, then place the remainder in a food processor or blender with the onion, ginger and half the chillies. Add 75ml/5 tbsp of the water and process to a smooth paste.

3 Heat the groundnut oil in a large frying pan, add the cumin seeds and cook for about 30 seconds.

4 Stir the coriander seeds, turmeric, chilli powder and ground cashew nuts in to the pan. Add the ginger and chilli paste and cook, stirring frequently, until the water begins to evaporate. Add the chopped tomatoes and stir-fry until the mixture begins to turn a red-brown colour.

5 Mix in the chickpeas and parsnips with the remaining water, 5ml/1 tsp salt and plenty of black pepper. Bring to the boil, stir, then simmer, uncovered, for 15–20 minutes, until the parsnips are completely tender. Reduce the liquid, if necessary, by boiling fiercely until it has thickened slightly.

> **Cook's tip**
>
> If you don't have the time to soak dried chickpeas, use a 400g/14oz can instead. Add the drained chickpeas 10 minutes after the parsnips are added in step 4.

6 Add the ground roasted cumin with more salt and/or lime juice to taste. Stir in the reserved garlic and green chilli, and cook for 1–2 minutes. Scatter the coriander leaves and toasted cashew nuts over and serve straight away with a dollop of natural yogurt.

Nutrition notes	
Per portion:	
Energy	480Kcals/2006kJ
Protein	17.1g
Fat	22.2g
saturated fat	3g
Carbohydrate	56.4g
Fibre	16.3g
Calcium	180.4mg
Folate	296µg
Vitamin B_{12}	0µg
Selenium	9.2µg
Iron	4.9mg
Zinc	2.9mg

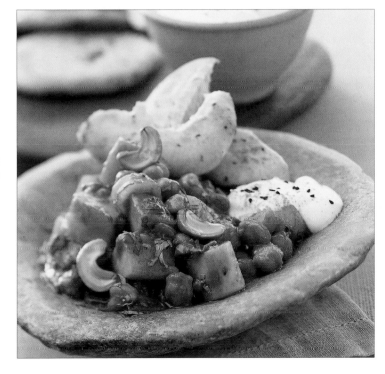

Spicy lamb with apricots and Indian rice

Perfect to serve in late pregnancy as lamb, split peas and dried apricots all provide lots of iron.

Serves 4

675g/1½lb lamb leg fillet, cubed
15ml/1 tbsp olive oil
1 onion, finely chopped
5ml/1 tsp ground coriander
10ml/2 tsp ground cumin
5ml/1 tsp fenugreek
2.5ml/½ tsp ground turmeric
pinch of cayenne pepper
1 cinnamon stick
120ml/4fl oz/½ cup chicken stock
175g/6oz/¾ cup ready-to-eat dried apricots,
   halved or quartered
salt and ground black pepper
fresh coriander (cilantro), to garnish

For the marinade
120ml/4fl oz/½ cup natural yogurt
15ml/1 tbsp sunflower oil
juice of ½ lemon
2.5cm/1in piece fresh root ginger, finely grated

For the rice
175g/6oz/¾ cup chana dhal or yellow split peas,
   soaked for 1–2 hours
225g/8oz/generous 1 cup basmati rice, soaked
   and drained
15ml/1 tbsp olive oil
1 large onion, finely sliced in rings
1 garlic clove, crushed
10ml/2 tsp grated fresh root ginger
60ml/4 tbsp natural yogurt
15ml/1 tbsp chopped fresh coriander (cilantro)

1 Make the marinade by blending together the yogurt, oil, lemon juice and ginger. Add the meat, stir to coat, then cover and leave in a cool place for 2–4 hours, or in the refrigerator overnight.

2 To make the rice, first put the chana dhal or split peas in a large pan, cover with boiling water and boil for 20 minutes, or until tender. Drain.

3 Cook the drained rice in boiling salted water for about 10 minutes until almost tender. Drain. Set aside.

4 Heat the olive oil in a frying pan and fry the onion for 5 minutes, or until golden. Transfer to a plate. Stir in the garlic and ginger and fry for a few seconds, then add the yogurt and cook for a few minutes, stirring. Add the cooked dhal or peas, the coriander, and salt to taste. Stir well, then remove from the heat and set aside. Preheat the oven to 180°C/350°F/ Gas 4.

5 Drain the meat, reserving the marinade. Heat the olive oil in a flameproof casserole and fry the onion for 3–4 minutes until soft. Add the spices and fry over a medium heat until they are sizzling.

6 Add the meat and fry until browned, then add the remaining marinade, and the chicken stock and apricots. Season well. Bring to the boil, then cover and cook in the oven for 45–55 minutes until the meat is tender.

7 Meanwhile, finish cooking the rice. Spoon the dhal mixture into a casserole and stir in the rice. Sprinkle with the onion rings. Cover with a double layer of foil, secured with the lid. Place in the oven 30 minutes before the lamb is ready. The rice and dhal should be tender but the grains should be separate. Serve the rice and spiced lamb together, garnished with the fresh coriander.

Nutrition notes	
Per portion:	
Energy	803Kcals/3356kJ
Protein	52.3g
Fat	24.8g
saturated fat	7.8g
Carbohydrate	96.3g
Fibre	6.9g
Calcium	158.7mg
Folate	36.6μg
Vitamin B$_{12}$	3.4μg
Selenium	4.6μg
Iron	7.3mg
Zinc	7.8mg

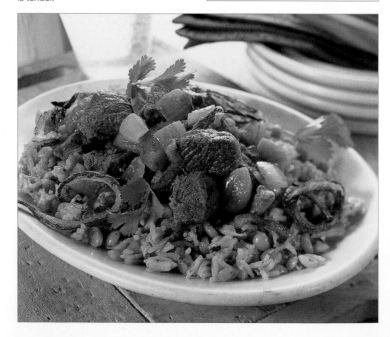

Lamb burgers with tomato relish

These spicy burgers are packed with iron, immune-boosting carotenoids and vitamin B$_{12}$.

Serves 4

25g/1oz/3 tbsp bulgur wheat
500g/1¼lb lean minced (ground) lamb
1 small red onion, finely chopped
2 garlic cloves, finely chopped
1 fresh green chilli, seeded and chopped
5ml/1 tsp ground toasted cumin seeds
15g/½oz/⅓ cup chopped parsley
30ml/2 tbsp chopped fresh mint
salt and ground black pepper
olive oil, for frying

For the relish
2 red (bell) peppers, halved and seeded
2 red onions, cut into 5mm/¼in thick slices
75–90ml/5–6 tbsp extra virgin olive oil
350g/12oz cherry tomatoes, chopped
½ fresh red or green chilli, seeded and finely
   chopped
30ml/2 tbsp chopped fresh mint
30ml/2 tbsp chopped fresh parsley
15ml/1 tbsp chopped fresh oregano
2.5ml/½ tsp ground toasted cumin seeds
juice of ½ lemon
caster (superfine) sugar, to taste

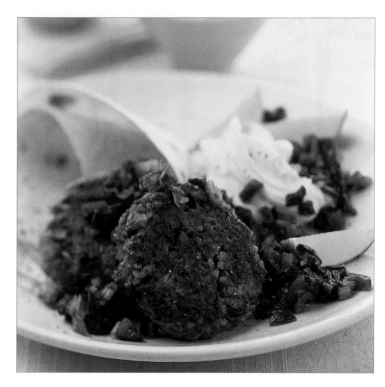

1 Pour 150ml/¼ pint/⅔ cup boiling water over the bulgur wheat in a bowl and leave to stand for 15 minutes, then drain in a sieve (strainer) lined with a clean dish towel. Squeeze out the excess moisture.

2 Place the bulgur wheat in a bowl and add the lamb, onion, garlic, chilli, cumin, parsley and mint. Mix together by hand, then season with 5ml/1 tsp salt and plenty of black pepper and mix again.

3 Form the mixture into eight small round burgers and set aside.

4 Grill (broil) the peppers, skin side up, until they blister and begin to char. Place in a bowl, cover and leave to stand for 10 minutes, then peel.

5 Meanwhile, brush the onions with 15ml/1 tbsp oil and grill for about 5 minutes on each side. Leave to cool.

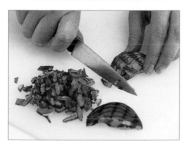

6 Chop the peppers and onions and place in a bowl with the tomatoes, chilli, herbs and cumin. Stir in 60ml/4 tbsp of the oil and 15ml/1 tbsp of the lemon juice. Season with salt, pepper and sugar and set aside for 25 minutes, then add more lemon juice, if needed.

7 Heat a heavy frying pan or ridged, cast-iron griddle over a high heat and grease lightly with olive oil. Cook the burgers for 6 minutes on each side, or until cooked through to your taste. Serve immediately, with the relish.

Nutrition notes	
Per portion:	
Energy	457Kcals/1910kJ
Protein	26.9g
Fat	31.2g
saturated fat	9.8g
Carbohydrate	18.5g
Fibre	4g
Calcium	67.5mg
Folate	57µg
Vitamin B$_{12}$	2.5µg
Selenium	3.8µg
Iron	3.1mg
Zinc	4.8mg

Beef and vegetable stir-fry

This superb mixture of peppers, full of antioxidants, and beef with iron and vitamin B_{12} offers a complete nutritional package in one dish.

Serves 4

225g/8oz rump (round) or sirloin steak
115g/4oz cellophane noodles, soaked for
   20 minutes in hot water to cover
4 Chinese dried mushrooms, soaked for
   30 minutes in warm water
25ml/1½ tbsp sunflower oil
2 eggs, separated
1 carrot, cut into matchsticks
1 onion, sliced
2 courgettes (zucchini), cut into sticks
½ red (bell) pepper, seeded and cut into strips
4 button (white) mushrooms, sliced
75g/3oz/1 cup beansprouts
15ml/1 tbsp light soy sauce
salt and ground black pepper
sliced spring onions (scallions) and sesame
   seeds, to garnish

For the marinade
15ml/1 tbsp granulated sugar
30ml/2 tbsp light soy sauce
45ml/3 tbsp sesame oil
4 spring onions (scallions), chopped
1 garlic clove, crushed
10ml/2 tsp crushed toasted sesame seeds

1 Freeze the steak until it is firm enough to cut into thin slices, then into 5cm/2in strips. Mix the ingredients for the marinade in a bowl and add the steak.

2 Drain the noodles and cook them in boiling water for 5 minutes. Drain again, then snip into short lengths. Drain the soaked mushrooms, cut off and discard the stems; slice the caps.

3 Heat 10ml/2 tsp oil in a small frying pan. Beat the egg yolks and pour into the pan. When set, slide on to a plate. Cook the egg whites until set. Cut both yolks and whites into diamond shapes and set aside for the garnish. Remove the beef strips from the marinade.

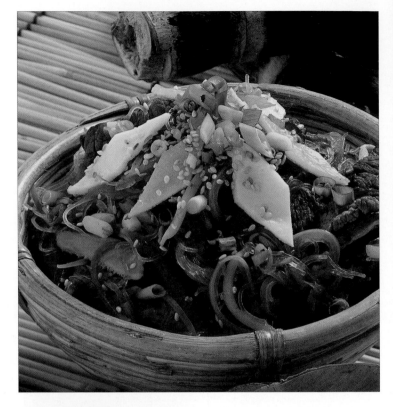

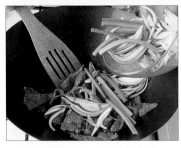

4 Heat the remaining oil in a wok or large frying pan and stir-fry the beef until it changes colour. Add the carrot matchsticks and the onion and stir-fry for 2 minutes, then add the other vegetables, tossing them over the heat until they are just cooked but still retaining their bite.

5 Add the noodles and season with soy sauce, salt and pepper. Cook for 1 minute. Serve, garnished with egg, spring onions and sesame seeds.

Nutrition notes	
Per portion:	
Energy	274Kcals/1145kJ
Protein	20.3g
Fat	7.4g
saturated fat	2.6g
Carbohydrate	31.1g
Fibre	2.6g
Calcium	58.6mg
Folate	73.5µg
Vitamin B_{12}	1.8µg
Selenium	12.8µg
Iron	3.4mg
Zinc	2.5mg

Soft corn tortillas with beef

These tortillas offer good supplies of fertility-boosting zinc, for pre-conception and iron during pregnancy, to counteract anaemia.

Makes 12

500g/1¼lb rump (round) steak, diced into
   1cm/½in pieces
2 garlic cloves, peeled and left whole
750ml/1¼ pints/3 cups beef stock
150g/5oz/1 cup masa harina
pinch of salt
120ml/4fl oz/½ cup warm water
7.5ml/1½ tsp dried oregano
2.5ml/½ tsp ground cumin
30ml/2 tbsp tomato purée (paste)
2.5ml/½ tsp granulated sugar
salt and ground black pepper
shredded lettuce and onion relish,
   to serve

3 Divide the dough into 12 small balls. Open a tortilla press and line both sides with clear film (plastic wrap). Put a ball of dough on the tortilla press and bring the top down to flatten the dough into a 5–6.5cm/ 2–2½in round. Flatten the remaining dough balls in the same way.

4 Heat a griddle or frying pan until hot. Cook each tortilla for about 20 seconds on each side, and then for another 20 seconds on the first side. Keep the tortillas warm and soft inside a slightly damp dish towel.

5 Add the oregano, cumin, tomato purée and sugar to the pan of beef, with just enough beef stock to keep the mixture moist. Cook gently for a few minutes.

6 Place a little of the lettuce on a warm tortilla. Top with a little filling and relish, fold in half and serve warm. Fill more tortillas in the same way.

Nutrition notes	
Per filled tortilla:	
Energy	103Kcals/430kJ
Protein	11.3g
Fat	3.2g
saturated fat	1.4g
Carbohydrate	6.9g
Fibre	0.1g
Calcium	7mg
Folate	6.1µg
Vitamin B_{12}	1µg
Selenium	3.5µg
Iron	1.1mg
Zinc	1.4mg

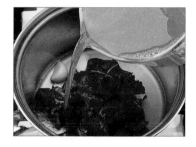

1 Put the diced beef and whole garlic cloves in a large pan and cover with the beef stock. Bring to the boil, lower the heat and simmer for 10–15 minutes, until the meat is tender. Using a slotted spoon, transfer the meat to a clean pan and set it aside. Reserve the stock.

2 Mix the masa harissa It in a large bowl. Add the warm water, a little at a time, to make a dough that can be worked into a ball. Knead this on a lightly floured surface for 3–4 minutes, until smooth, then wrap in clear film and set aside for 1 hour.

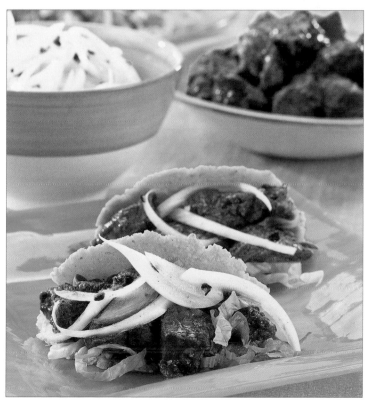

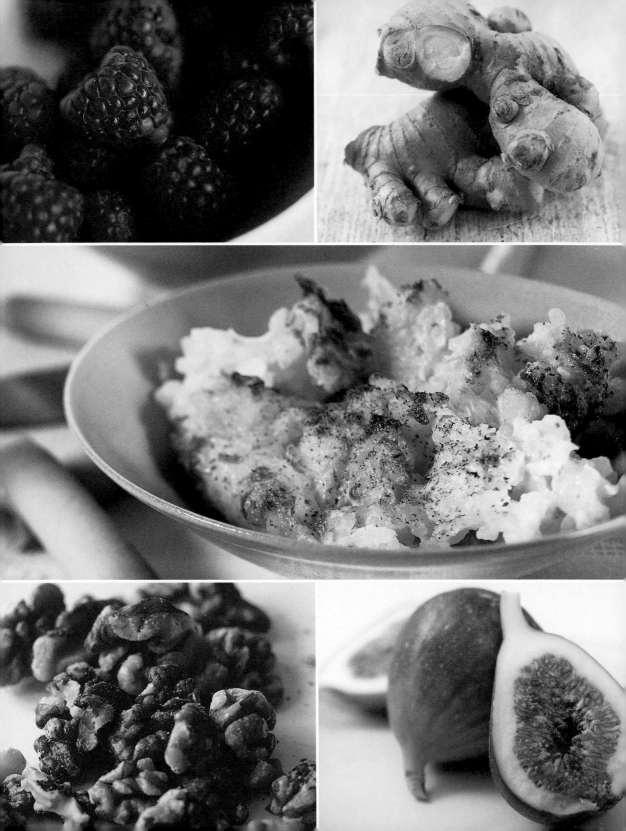

desserts
and bakes

You should be eating nutritious foods for optimum fertility
and a healthy pregnancy, but there's no need to miss out fresh
fruit desserts, such as Summer Pudding and Papaya Baked with
Ginger. Breads, cakes and cookies that contain wholegrain flours,
nuts and dried fruits are also full of valuable nutrients, and these
carbohydrate-rich snacks are ideal for fending off morning
sickness and chocolate cravings later in pregnancy.

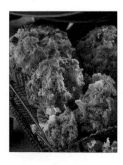
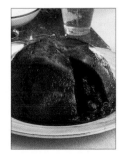
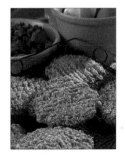

Summer pudding

This classic fruit dessert is low in fat and rich in vitamin C.

Serves 4

8 × 1cm/½in-thick slices of day-old white bread, crusts removed
800g/1¾lb/8–9 cups mixed soft fruits, such as strawberries, raspberries, blackcurrants, redcurrants and blueberries
50g/2oz/¼ cup caster (superfine) sugar
low-fat crème fraîche or fromage frais, to serve

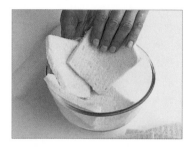

1 Trim a slice of bread to fit in the base of a 1.2 litre/2 pint/5 cup ovenproof bowl, then trim another 5–6 slices to line the sides of the bowl.

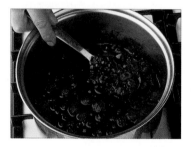

2 Place all the fruit in a pan with the sugar. Cook over a low heat for 4–5 minutes until the juices begin to run – it will not be necessary to add any water.

3 Allow the mixture to cool slightly, then spoon the berries and enough of their juices to moisten into the bread-lined bowl. Save any leftover juice.

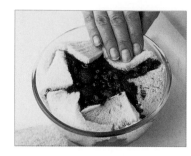

4 Fold any excess bread that extends above the fruit mixture into the centre. Cover the top of the pudding with the remaining bread slices, trimming them neatly to fit. Place a small plate or saucer directly on top of the pudding, fitting it inside the bowl.

5 Weight the plate or saucer down with a 1kg or 2lb weight if you have one, or use two full food cans.

6 Chill the pudding for at least 8 hours or overnight. To serve, run a knife between the pudding and the bowl and turn it out on a plate. Spoon the reserved juices over. Serve with crème fraîche or fromage frais.

Nutrition notes	
Per portion:	
Energy	182Kcals/761kJ
Protein	5.2g
Fat	1g
saturated fat	0g
Carbohydrate	40.2g
Fibre	2.2g
Calcium	75.1mg
Folate	39.4µg
Vitamin B$_{12}$	0.6µg
Selenium	13.8µg
Iron	1.5mg
Zinc	0.5mg

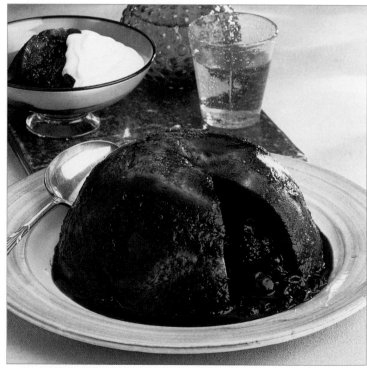

Melon trio with ginger thins

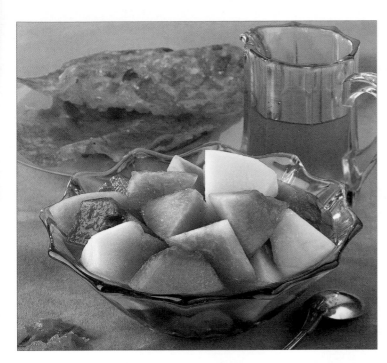

The ginger in this refreshing fruit salad will help to settle the stomach. Eat the salad for dessert, or try it for breakfast.

Serves 4

¼ watermelon
½ honeydew melon
½ Charentais melon
60ml/4 tbsp syrup from a jar of stem (crystallized) ginger

For the ginger thins

25g/1oz/2 tbsp unsalted butter
25g/1oz/2 tbsp caster (superfine) sugar
5ml/1 tsp clear honey
25g/1oz/¼ cup plain (all-purpose) flour
25g/1oz/¼ cup luxury mixed glacé (candied) fruit, finely chopped
1 piece stem (crystallized) ginger in syrup, drained and finely chopped
30ml/2 tbsp flaked (sliced) almonds

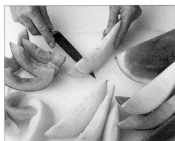

1 Remove the seeds from the melons, cut them into wedges, then slice off the rind. Cut all the flesh into chunks and mix in a bowl. Stir in the ginger syrup, cover and chill until ready to serve.

Variation

If you're feeling run down, substitute cantaloupe for the honeydew melon for an immune-boosting dose of carotenoids.

---

2 Meanwhile, make the ginger thins. Preheat the oven to 180°C/350°F/ Gas 4. Melt the butter, sugar and honey in a small pan. Remove from the heat and stir in the remaining ingredients.

3 Line a baking sheet with baking parchment. Space four spoonfuls of the mixture on the paper at regular intervals, leaving plenty of room for spreading. Flatten the mixture slightly into rounds and bake for 15 minutes or until the tops are golden brown.

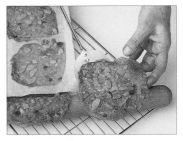

4 Let the thins cool on the baking sheet for 1 minute, then lift each one in turn, using a spatula, and drape over a rolling pin to cool and harden. Repeat with the remaining ginger mixture to make eight thins in all. Leave to cool completely on a wire rack.

5 Serve the chilled melon salad with the ginger thins.

Nutrition notes	
Per portion:	
Energy	286Kcals/1195kJ
Protein	3.5g
Fat	10.3g
saturated fat	3.7g
Carbohydrate	47.9g
Fibre	1.2g
Calcium	49.9mg
Folate	7.8µg
Vitamin B$_{12}$	0.3µg
Selenium	0.6µg
Iron	1.3mg
Zinc	0.8mg

Papaya with spiced ginger

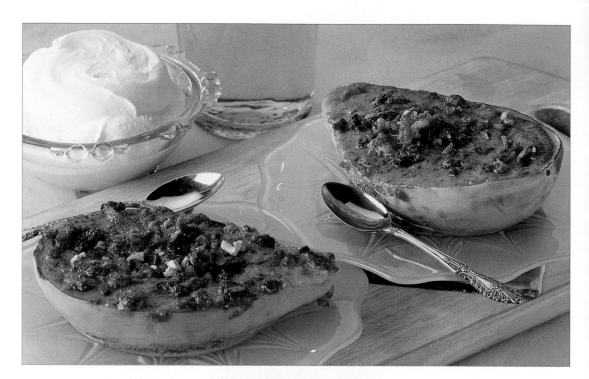

This is the perfect pregnancy dessert. Not only does it taste delicious, but the fresh papaya and ginger will help to settle your stomach and the potassium-rich pistachio nuts are good for easing muscle cramps.

Serves 4

2 ripe papayas
2 pieces stem (crystallized) ginger in syrup, drained, plus 15ml/1 tbsp syrup from the jar
8 amaretti or other dessert cookies, coarsely crushed
45ml/3 tbsp raisins
shredded rind and juice of 1 lime
25g/1oz/¼ cup pistachio nuts, chopped
15ml/1 tbsp light muscovado (molasses) sugar
60ml/4 tbsp crème fraîche, plus extra to serve

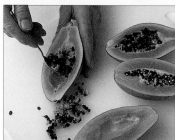

1 Preheat the oven to 200°C/400°F/ Gas 6. Cut the papayas in half and scoop out their seeds. Place the halves in a baking dish and set aside. Cut the stem ginger into fine matchsticks.

2 Make the filling. Combine the crushed amaretti, stem ginger matchsticks and raisins in a bowl. Stir in the lime rind and juice, and two-thirds of the nuts, then add the sugar and the crème fraîche. Mix well.

3 Fill the papaya halves with the amaretti and ginger mixture and drizzle with the ginger syrup. Sprinkle the remaining nuts over the top. Bake for about 25 minutes or until tender. Serve on dessert plates with extra crème fraîche.

Nutrition notes	
Per portion:	
Energy	399Kcals/1667kJ
Protein	3.4g
Fat	20.2g
saturated fat	4.9g
Carbohydrate	53.8g
Fibre	3.9g
Calcium	70.5mg
Folate	8.9µg
Vitamin B$_{12}$	0.1µg
Selenium	1.7µg
Iron	1.8mg
Zinc	0.5mg

Spiced pineapple with papaya sauce

Cinnamon and ginger flavour this vitamin C-rich dessert.

Serves 6

1 sweet pineapple
melted butter, for greasing and brushing
2 pieces drained stem (crystallized) ginger in
    syrup, cut into matchsticks, plus 30ml/2 tbsp
    syrup from the jar
30ml/2 tbsp demerara (raw) sugar
pinch of ground cinnamon
fresh mint sprigs, to decorate

For the sauce
1 ripe papaya, peeled and seeded
175ml/6fl oz/¾ cup apple juice

1 Peel the pineapple and remove the eyes. Cut it crossways into six slices, each about 2.5cm/1in thick.

2 Line a baking sheet with foil, rolling up the sides to make a rim and grease the foil lightly with melted butter. Preheat the grill (broiler).

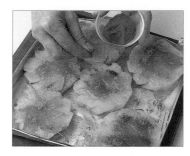

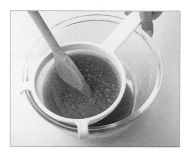

3 Arrange the pineapple slices on the lined baking sheet. Brush with melted butter, then scatter the ginger matchsticks, sugar and cinnamon on top. Drizzle over the syrup. Grill (broil) for 5–7 minutes or until the slices are golden and lightly charred on top.

4 Meanwhile, make the sauce. Cut a few slices from the papaya and set aside, then purée the rest with the apple juice in a blender or food processor.

5 Press the papaya and apple purée through a strainer placed over a bowl. Drain off any juices from the baking sheet on which the pineapple was cooked, and stir these gently into the purée.

6 Place a pineapple slice on each dessert plate and drizzle a little of the sauce over each. Decorate with the reserved papaya slices and the frest mint sprigs.

Cook's tip

If you're past your due date, then try eating a raw version of this dish, as the enzyme bromelain, found in uncooked pineapple, is said to help bring on labour.

Nutrition notes

Per portion:

Energy	90Kcals/376kJ
Protein	0.4g
Fat	1.5g
saturated fat	0.9g
Carbohydrate	20.1g
Fibre	1.1g
Calcium	18.7mg
Folate	3.1µg
Vitamin B$_{12}$	0µg
Selenium	0µg
Iron	0.3mg
Zinc	0.1mg

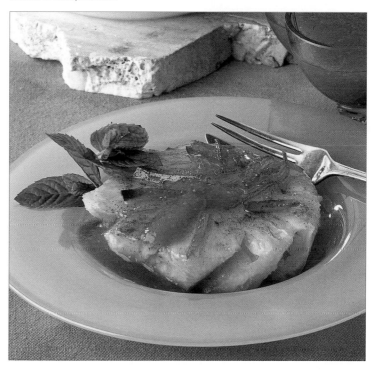

Soufléed rice pudding

Rich in calcium, this light pudding can be eaten as a snack in the late stages of pregnancy or as a meal substitute early on, when you may be feeling queasy.

Serves 4

65g/2½oz/⅓ cup short grain pudding rice
45ml/3 tbsp clear honey
750ml/1¼ pints/3 cups skimmed milk
1 vanilla pod (bean), split with a sharp knife, or 2.5ml/½ tsp vanilla extract
butter, for greasing
2 egg whites
5ml/1 tsp freshly grated nutmeg
biscuits or cookies, to serve (optional)

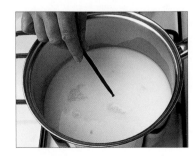

1 Place the rice, honey and milk in a heavy or non-stick pan, and bring the milk to just below boiling point, watching it very closely to prevent it from boiling over. Add the vanilla pod to the milk, if using.

2 Reduce the heat to the lowest setting and cover the pan. Leave to cook for about 1–1¼ hours, stirring occasionally to prevent sticking, until most of the liquid has been absorbed.

3 Remove the vanilla pod from the pan or, if using vanilla essence, add this to the rice mixture now. Preheat the oven to 220°C/425°F/Gas 7. Grease a 1 litre/1¾ pint/4 cup baking dish with butter.

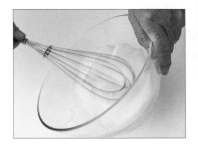

4 Whisk the egg whites until holding soft peaks, then carefully fold them into the rice and milk mixture. Tip the mixture into the baking dish and spread evenly.

5 Sprinkle with grated nutmeg and bake for 15–20 minutes, until the rice pudding has risen well and the surface is golden brown. Serve hot, with biscuits or cookies, if you like.

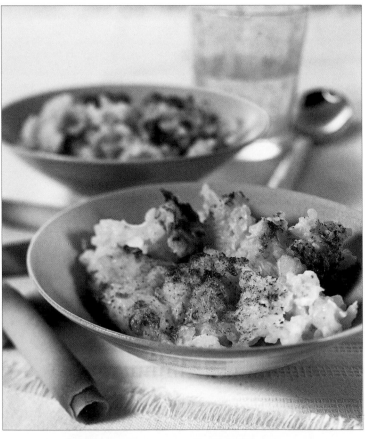

Nutrition notes	
Per portion:	
Energy	166Kcals/694kJ
Protein	9g
Fat	0.4g
saturated fat	0.2g
Carbohydrate	32.2g
Fibre	0g
Calcium	279mg
Folate	13.3µg
Vitamin B_{12}	0.7µg
Selenium	2.9µg
Iron	0.4mg
Zinc	1.3mg

Apricot panettone pudding

The apricots in this rich pudding provide immune-boosting betacarotene and iron for later in pregnancy. The nuts supply fertility-promoting vitamin E.

Serves 6

unsalted butter, for greasing
350g/12oz panettone, sliced thickly then cut into triangles
25g/1oz/¼ cup pecan nuts
75g/3oz/⅓ cup ready-to-eat dried apricots, chopped
550ml/18fl oz/2½ cups semi-skimmed (low-fat) milk
5ml/1 tsp vanilla essence (extract)
1 large egg, beaten
30ml/2 tbsp maple syrup
2.5ml/½ tsp grated nutmeg, plus extra for sprinkling
demerara (raw) sugar, for sprinkling
low-fat crème fraîche, to serve

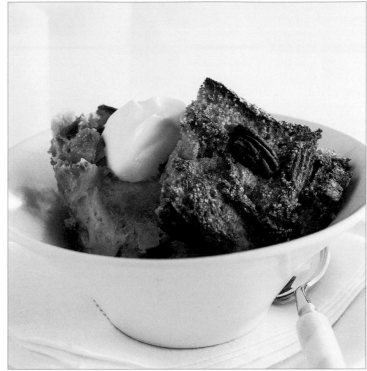

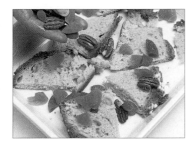

1 Grease a 1 litre/1¾ pint/4 cup baking dish. Arrange half the panettone slices in the base of the dish, scatter over half the pecan nuts and all the dried apricots, then add another layer of panettone on top, spreading it as evenly as you can.

2 Pour the milk into a medium pan and add the vanilla essence. Warm the milk over a medium heat until it just simmers. In a large jug (pitcher), mix together the beaten egg and maple syrup, grate in the nutmeg, then whisk in the hot milk. Preheat the oven to 200°C/400°F/Gas 6.

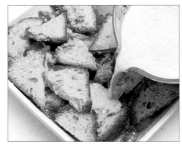

3 Pour the milk mixture over the panettone, lightly pressing down each slice so it is submerged. Set aside for at least 10 minutes.

Cook's tip
If you can't find panettone, use a similar light fruit bread.

4 Scatter the reserved pecan nuts over the top of the pudding and sprinkle with the sugar and nutmeg. Bake for 40 minutes until risen and golden. Serve with crème fraîche.

Nutrition notes

Per portion:

Energy	269Kcals/1124kJ
Protein	9.2g
Fat	9.8g
saturated fat	2.3g
Carbohydrate	38.6g
Fibre	0.9g
Calcium	167mg
Folate	23.7µg
Vitamin B$_{12}$	0.6µg
Selenium	3µg
Iron	1.7mg
Zinc	1.2mg

Double-ginger cake

This gingery tea bread is great at any time, but is particularly good first thing for those who are suffering from morning sickness.

Serves 8-10

3 eggs
225g/8oz/generous 1 cup caster (superfine) sugar
250ml/8fl oz/1 cup sunflower oil
5ml/1 tsp vanilla essence (extract)
15ml/1 tbsp syrup from a jar of stem (crystallized) ginger
225g/8oz courgettes (zucchini), grated
2.5cm/1in piece fresh root ginger, peeled and grated
350g/12oz/3 cups unbleached plain (all-purpose) flour
5ml/1 tsp baking powder
pinch of salt
5ml/1 tsp ground cinnamon
2 pieces stem (crystallized) ginger, drained and finely chopped
15ml/1 tbsp demerara (raw) sugar

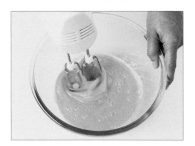

1 Preheat the oven to 190°C/375°F/ Gas 5. Beat together the eggs and sugar until light and fluffy. Slowly beat in the oil until the mixture forms a batter. Mix in the vanilla essence and ginger syrup, then stir in the courgettes and fresh ginger.

2 Sift together the flour, baking powder and salt into a large bowl. Add the cinnamon and mix well, then stir the dried ingredients into the courgette mixture.

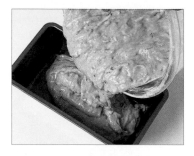

3 Lightly grease a 900g/2lb loaf tin (pan) and pour, then scrape in the courgette mixture, making sure it fills the corners. Smooth and level the top.

4 Mix together the chopped stem ginger and demerara sugar in a small bowl, then sprinkle evenly over the surface.

5 Bake for 1 hour or until a skewer comes out clean when inserted. Cool in the tin for 20 minutes, then turn out on to a wire rack.

Nutrition notes	
Per portion:	
Energy	409Kcals/1710kJ
Protein	5.7g
Fat	20.8g
saturated fat	2.7g
Carbohydrate	53.3g
Fibre	1.3g
Calcium	66.6mg
Folate	27.4µg
Vitamin B_{12}	0.4µg
Selenium	3.4µg
Iron	1.2mg
Zinc	0.5mg

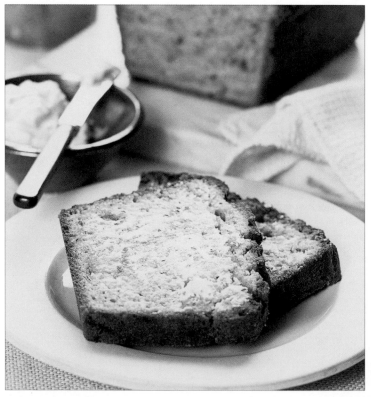

Yogurt and fig cake

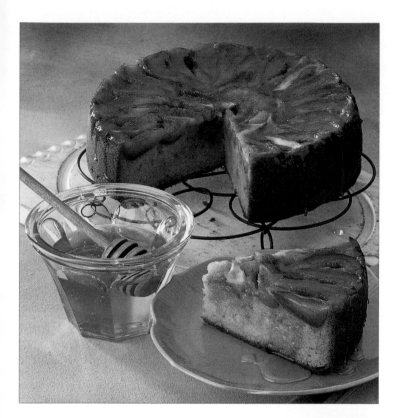

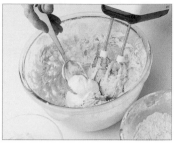

3 Sift together the dry ingredients. Add a little to the creamed butter and sugar mixture, beat well, then beat in a spoonful of the yogurt. Repeat this process until all the dry ingredients and yogurt have been incorporated.

4 Whisk the egg whites in a grease-free bowl until they form stiff peaks. Stir half the whites into the cake mixture to loosen it slightly, then gently fold in the remaining whites using a large spatula or spoon.

5 Pour the mixture over the figs in the tin (pan), then bake for about 1¼ hours or until golden and a skewer inserted in the centre comes out clean.

6 Turn the cake out on to a wire rack, then peel off the lining paper and leave to cool. Drizzle the figs with extra honey before serving.

This high-fibre cake contains useful amounts of calcium.

Serves 6-8

6 firm fresh figs, thickly sliced
45ml/3 tbsp clear honey, plus extra for glazing
   cooked figs
200g/7oz/scant 1 cup butter, softened
175g/6oz/¾ cup caster (superfine) sugar
grated rind of 1 lemon
grated rind of 1 orange
4 eggs, separated
225g/8oz/2 cups plain (all-purpose) flour
5ml/1 tsp baking powder
5ml/1 tsp bicarbonate of soda
   (baking soda)
250ml/8fl oz/1 cup thick natural (plain) yogurt

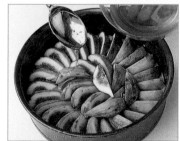

1 Preheat the oven to 180°C/350°F/ Gas 4. Grease a 23cm/9in round cake tin (pan) and line with baking parchment. Arrange the figs over the base and drizzle with honey.

2 In a large bowl, cream the butter and sugar with the citrus rinds, then beat in the egg yolks.

Nutrition notes	
Per portion:	
Energy	467Kcals/1952kJ
Protein	8.8g
Fat	24.5g
saturated fat	14.8g
Carbohydrate	56.8g
Fibre	1.5g
Calcium	138mg
Folate	26.8μg
Vitamin B$_{12}$	0.9μg
Selenium	4.9μg
Iron	1.4mg
Zinc	1mg

Date and apple muffins

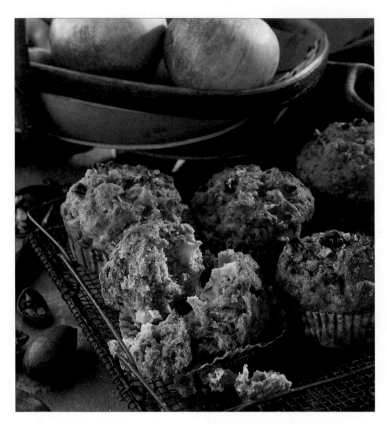

These high-fibre muffins contain useful amounts of zinc.

Makes 12

150g/5oz/1¼ cups self-raising wholemeal (whole-wheat) flour
150g/5oz/1¼ cups self-raising (self-rising) white flour
5ml/1 tsp ground cinnamon
5ml/1 tsp baking powder
25g/1oz/2 tbsp sunflower margarine
75g/3oz/½ cup light muscovado (molasses) sugar
250ml/8fl oz/1 cup apple juice
30ml/2 tbsp pear and apple spread
1 egg, lightly beaten
1 eating apple, finely chopped
75g/3oz/½cup chopped dates
15ml/1 tbsp chopped pecan nuts

1 Preheat the oven to 200°C/400°F/ Gas 6. Arrange 12 paper cases in a deep muffin tray (pan).

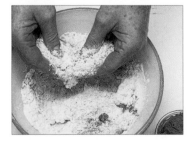

2 Put the wholemeal flour in a mixing bowl. Sift in the white flour with the cinnamon and baking powder. Rub in the margarine until the mixture resembles breadcrumbs. Stir in the sugar.

3 Stir a little of the apple juice into the pear and apple spread until it forms a smooth paste. Mix in the remaining apple juice, then mix into the rubbed-in mixture with the beaten egg.

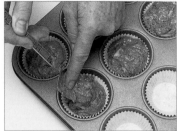

4 Add the chopped apple and dates. Mix quickly until just combined, then divide among the muffin cases.

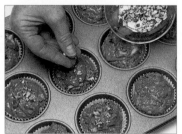

5 Sprinkle the chopped pecans over the top of the mixture. Bake for about 20–25 minutes, until well risen and golden brown. Serve warm.

Nutrition notes	
Per portion:	
Energy	173Kcals/723kJ
Protein	3.8g
Fat	3.6g
saturated fat	0.6g
Carbohydrate	33.7g
Fibre	1.9g
Calcium	33.5mg
Folate	14.4µg
Vitamin B$_{12}$	0.13µg
Selenium	7.9µg
Iron	1mg
Zinc	0.6mg

Malted oat cookies

The oats in these crisp cookies provide vitamin E, as well as soluble fibre, which is very important during pregnancy.

Makes 18

175g/6oz/1½ cups rolled oats
75g/3oz/½ cup light muscovado (molasses) sugar
1 egg
60ml/4 tbsp sunflower or vegetable oil
30ml/2 tbsp malt extract

1 Preheat the oven to 190°C/375°F/ Gas 5. Lightly grease two baking sheets. Mix the rolled oats and brown sugar in a bowl, breaking up any lumps in the sugar. Add the egg, sunflower oil and malt extract, mix well, then set the mixture aside to soak for 15 minutes.

Variation

Try replacing 25g/1oz/¼ cup of the rolled oats with ground Brazil nuts for a healthy dose of selenium

---

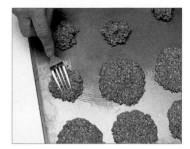

2 Using a teaspoon, place small heaps of the mixture well apart on the prepared baking sheets. Press the heaps into 7.5cm/3in rounds with the back of a dampened fork.

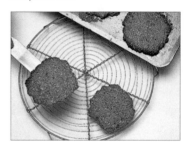

3 Bake the biscuits in the oven for 10–15 minutes, until golden brown. Leave to cool on the baking sheets for 1 minute, then remove with a palette knife or metal spatula and cool on a wire rack.

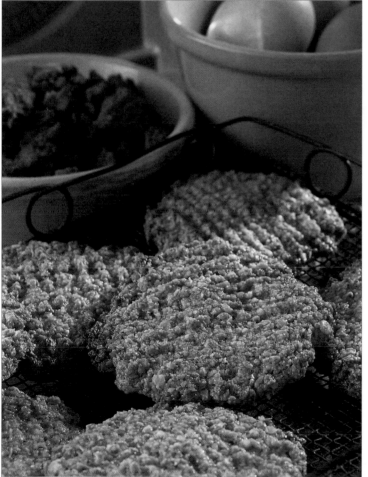

Nutrition notes	
Per biscuit:	
Energy	81Kcals/338kJ
Protein	1.6g
Fat	3.6g
saturated fat	0.4g
Carbohydrate	11.3g
Fibre	0.7g
Calcium	9.4mg
Folate	7.4µg
Vitamin B_{12}	0.09µg
Selenium	0.6µg
Iron	0.5mg
Zinc	0.4mg

Fruit and saffron bread

This spiced tea bread contains useful amounts of vitamin E for fertility and plenty of calcium for pregnancy and breastfeeding.

Makes 2 loaves

300ml/½ pint/1¼ cups milk
2.5ml/½ tsp saffron strands
400g/14oz/3½ cups strong white bread
    flour
25g/1oz fresh yeast, crumbled, or 15ml/1 tbsp
    dried active yeast
50g/2oz/½ cup ground almonds
2.5ml/½ tsp grated nutmeg
2.5ml/½ tsp ground cinnamon
50g/2oz/¼ cup caster (superfine) sugar
2.5ml/½ tsp salt
75g/3oz/6 tbsp butter, softened
50g/2oz/⅓ cup sultanas
50g/2oz/¼ cup currants

For the glaze

30ml/2 tbsp milk
15ml/1 tbsp caster (superfine) sugar

1 Lightly grease two 900g/2lb loaf tins (pans). Heat half the milk in a small pan until almost boiling.

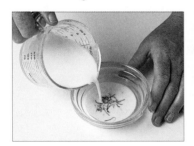

2 Place the saffron strands in a small heatproof bowl and pour over the milk. Stir gently, then leave to infuse for 30 minutes. Heat the remaining milk in the same pan until it is just lukewarm.

3 Place 50g/2oz/½ cup of the flour in a bowl, stir in the yeast and the lukewarm milk. Mix well, then leave for 15 minutes until the liquid is frothy.

4 Mix the remaining flour, ground almonds, spices, sugar and salt in a bowl and make a well in the centre. Add the saffron infusion, yeast mixture and butter and mix to a soft dough.

5 Turn the dough on to a floured surface and knead for 5 minutes. Place in an oiled bowl, cover with oiled clear film (plastic wrap) and leave to rise, in a warm place, for 1½–2 hours, or until doubled in bulk.

6 Tip the dough on to a floured surface and knock back (punch down), then knead in the dried fruit. Shape into two loaves and place in the tins. Cover with oiled clear film and leave to rise, for 1½ hours, or until the dough reaches the top of the tins.

7 Meanwhile, preheat the oven to 220°C/425°F/Gas 7. Bake the loaves for 10 minutes, then reduce the heat to 190°C/375°F/Gas 5 and bake for about 15–20 minutes or until golden.

8 To make the glaze. heat the milk and sugar in a small pan, stirring with a wooden spoon until the sugar dissolves. When the loaves come out of the oven, brush with the glaze immediately. Leave in the tins for 5 minutes, then turn on to a wire rack and set aside to cool slightly. Serve warm or toasted.

Nutrition notes	
Per loaf:	
Energy	1414Kcals/5910kJ
Protein	30.5g
Fat	49.8g
saturated fat	23.6g
Carbohydrate	225g
Fibre	9g
Calcium	567.4mg
Folate	72.5µg
Vitamin B$_{12}$	0.6µg
Selenium	10.5µg
Iron	5.8mg
Zinc	2.8mg

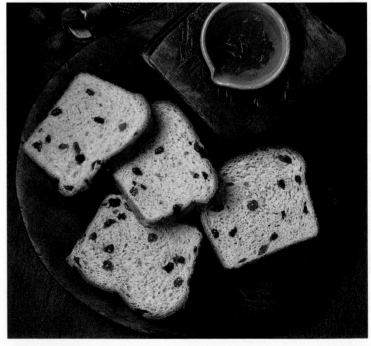

Walnut bread

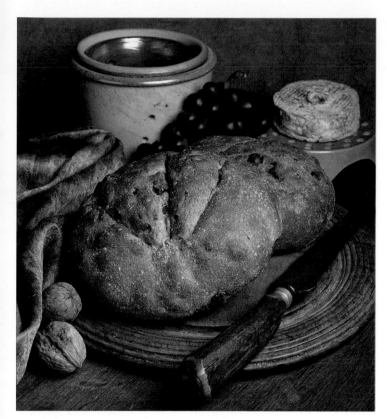

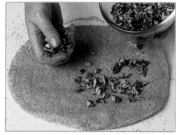

4 Place in a lightly oiled bowl, cover with oiled clear film (plastic wrap) and leave to rise in a warm place for about 1 hour, or until doubled in bulk.

5 Knock back (punch down) the dough on a floured surface, then flatten. Sprinkle over the nuts and gently press in. Roll up the dough and return it to the bowl. Cover and leave in a warm place for 30 minutes.

6 Divide the dough in half and shape each piece into a ball. Place on the baking sheets, cover with lightly oiled clear film (plastic wrap) and leave to rise in a warm place for 45 minutes, or until the loaves have doubled in size.

7 Preheat the oven to 220°C/425°F/ Gas 7. Slash the top of each loaf three times. Bake for about 35 minutes, or until the loaves sound hollow when tapped on the base. Cool on wire racks.

Walnuts contain useful amounts of omega-3 and omega-6 fatty acids, which are needed for your baby's growing brain.

Makes 2 loaves

50g/2oz/¼cup butter
350g/12oz/3 cups wholemeal
  (whole-wheat) bread flour
115g/4oz/1 cup strong white bread flour
15ml/1 tbsp light brown muscovado (molasses)
  sugar
7.5ml/1½tsp salt
20g/¾oz fresh yeast or 10ml/2 tsp active dried
  yeast
275ml/9fl oz/generous 1 cup lukewarm milk
175g/6oz/1½ cups walnut pieces

1 Lightly grease two baking sheets. Place the butter in a small pan and heat until melted and starting to turn brown, then set aside to cool. Mix the flours, sugar and salt in a large bowl and make a well in the centre. Cream the yeast with half the milk. Add to the centre of the flour with the remaining milk.

2 Pour the cool melted butter through a fine strainer into the centre of the flour so that it joins the liquids already there. Using your hand, mix the liquids together in the bowl and gradually mix in small quantities of the flour to make a batter. Continue until the mixture forms a moist dough.

3 Knead the dough on a lightly floured surface for 6–8 minutes.

Nutrition notes	
Per loaf:	
Energy	1588Kcals/6638kJ
Protein	45.2g
Fat	87.2g
saturated fat	20.6g
Carbohydrate	166g
Fibre	20.6g
Calcium	398mg
Folate	178.4µg
Vitamin B$_{12}$	0.6µg
Selenium	113µg
Iron	10.6mg
Zinc	8.4mg

Useful addresses

UK

Bliss
2nd Floor, Chapter House
18-20 Crucifix Lane
London SE1 3JW
tel: 020 7378 1122
www.bliss.org.uk
support for parents of premature babies

Foresight
The Association for the Promotion of
Preconceptual Care
3 Lower Queens Road
Clevedon, BS21 6LX
tel: 01275 878953
www.foresight-preconception.org.uk

The Human Fertilisation and Embryology
Authority
103-105 Bunhill Road
London EC1Y 8HF
tel: 020 7291 8200
www.hfea.gov.uk/ForPatients

Infertility Network UK
Charter House
43 St Leonard's Road
Bexhill-on-Sea, TN40 1JA
tel: 0800 008 7464
www.infertilitynetworkuk.com

La Leche League
129a Middleton Boulevard
Wollaton Park
Nottingham NBG8 1FW
tel 0845 120 2918
www.laleche.org.uk
Breastfeeding support

Miscarriage Association
17 Wentworth Terrace
Wakefield WF1 3QW
tel: 01924 200799
www.miscarriageassociation.org.uk

The Multiple Births Foundation
Queen Charlotte's & Chelsea Hospital
Du Cane Road, London W12 0HS
tel: 020 3313 3519
www.multiplebirths.org.uk

National Childbirth Trust
Alexandra House
Oldham Terrace
Acton, London W3 6NH
tel: 0300 330 0700
www.nct.org.uk
Breastfeeding and postnatal problems

The National Institute of
Medical Herbalists
Clover House
James Court, South Street
Exeter EX1 1EE
tel: 01392 426022
www.nimh.org.uk

Relate
tel: 0845 1304010
www.relate.org.uk
Relationship counselling

Royal College of Obstetricians
and Gynaecologists
27 Sussex Place
London NW1 4RG
tel: 020 7772 6200
www.rcog.org.uk

The School of Meditation
158 Holland Park Avenue
London W11 4UH
tel: 020 7603 6116
www.schoolofmeditation.org

Twins and Multiple Birth Association
(TAMBA)
Manor House, Church Hill
Aldershot GU12 4JU
tel 01252 332344
www.tamba.org.uk

USA

American Holistic Medical Association
5313 Colorado Street
Duluth, NMN 55804
tel: 218 525 5651
www.aihm.org

American Institute of
Hypnotherapy
1805 E Garry Avenue
Suite 100, Santa Ana CA 92705
tel: 714 261 6400
www.aih.cc

American Massage Therapy Association
500 Davis Street, Suite 900
Evanston, IL 60201-4695
tel: 847 864 0123
www.amtamassage.org

American Osteopathic
Association
142 East Ontario Street
Chicago IL 60611
tel: 312 202 8000
www.osteopathic.org

American Red Cross
2025 E Street, NW
Washington DC 20006
tel: 202 303 4498
www.redcross.org

Food Allergy Initiative
7925 Jones Branch Drive
Suite 1100
McLean, VA22102
tel: 703 691 3179
www.foodallergy.org

National Association of
Childbearing Centers
3123 Gottschall Road
Perkiomenville PA 18074
tel: 215 234 8068
www.birthcenters.org

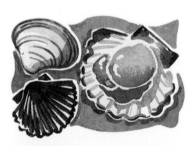

National Organization of Mothers
of Twins
PO Box 700860
Plymouth
Michigan 48170-0955
www.nomotc.org

National Women's Health Network
1413 K Street NW, 4th Floor
Washington DC 20005
tel: 202 682 2640
www.nwhn.org

Resolve (fertility problems)
The National Infertility Association
7918 Jones Branch Road, Suite 300
McLean VA 22102
tel: 703 556 7172
www.resolve.org

CANADA

Canadian Examining Board of
Health Care Practitioners Inc
658 Danforth Avenue
Suite 204, Toronto
Ontario M4J 5B9
tel: 416 466 9755
www.canadianexaminingboard.com

Canadian Women's Health
Network
Suite 203, 419 Graham Avenue
Winnipeg, Manitoba R3C 0M3
tel: 204 942 5500
www.cwhn.ca

Infertility Network
160 Pickering Street
Toronto, Ontario M4E 3J7
tel: 416 691 3611
www.infertilitynetwork.org

Multiple Births Canada
tel: 612 834 8946
www.multiplebirthscanada.org

AUSTRALIA

Austprem
www.austprem.org.au
Internet-based support for parents of
preterm babies

Australian Breastfeeding Association
1818 Malvern Road
East Malvern
Victoria 3145
tel: 03 9885 0855
www.breastfeeding.asn.au
Telephone numbers of breastfeeding
counsellors are posted on the website.

Complementary Medicine Association
Suite 14b
5 Michigan Drive
Oxenford QLD 4210
tel: 07 5580 5990
www.cma.asn.au

The Australian Multiple Births Association
(AMBA)
Po Box 105
Coogee, NSW 2034
tel: 1300 886 499
www.amba.org.au

Australian Women's Health Network
PO Box 188
Drysdale Vic 3222
www.awhn.org.au
Fertility Society of Australia
119 Buckhurst Street
South Melbourne, VIC 3205
tel: 3 9645 6359
www.fertilitysociety.com.au

NEW ZEALAND

The New Zealand Health
Information Network
PO Box 337
Christchurch 8015
tel: 03 980 4646
www.nzhealth.net.nz

Fertility New Zealand
PO Box 28262
Remuera, Auckland 1541
tel: 0800 333 306
www.fertilitynz.ord.nz

New Zealand Multiple Birth Association
PO Box 1258
Wellington
New Zealand
tel: 0800 489 467
www.multiples.org.nz

Early Buds
Early Buds
1/B Waiwhero Street
Mangakakahi, Rotorua 3015
tel: 027 348 8433
www.earlybuds.org.nz
Support for parents of premature and
poorly babies

Safekids Aotearoa
PO Box 26488
Epsom, Auckland 1344
tel: 9 630 9955
www.safekids.org.nz

SOUTH AFRICA

www.activebirth.co.za

African Health Anthology
www.nisc.co.za

WEBSITES

www.bygpub.com
www.babyfriendly.org.uk
www.talk-about-twins.com
www.tripletconnection.org

ACKNOWLEDGEMENTS
The author would like to thank the
following for their help and advice:
The British Nutrition Foundation,
Foresight, Greenpeace, Dr Michel
Odent, Pesticides Action Network,
and The Soil Association.

Index

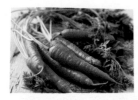